THE YOGA MASTERS SERIES

The Yoga Masters Series offers the timeless wisdom of essential yoga practices for the contemporary seeker.

BOOKS IN THE SERIES

Mantra

Mudrā

Prāṇa

Śavāsana

prāṇa

THE PRACTICE OF BODY, MIND, AND BREATH

Prasad Rangnekar

SHAMBHALA

Shambhala Publications, Inc.
2129 13th Street
Boulder, Colorado 80302
www.shambhala.com

Cover art: mmalkani/Shutterstock,
imaamut 027/Shutterstock, and renko_art/Shutterstock
Cover design: Daniel Urban-Brown
Interior design: Anna Becker

9 8 7 6 5 4 3 2 1

First Edition
Printed in the United States of America

Shambhala Publications makes every effort
to print on acid-free, recycled paper.
Shambhala Publications is distributed worldwide
by Penguin Random House, Inc., and its subsidiaries.

LIBRARY OF CONGRESS CATALOGING-IN-PUBLICATION DATA
Names: Rangnekar, Prasad author
Title: Prāṇa: the practice of body, mind, and breath / Prasad Rangnekar.
Description: First edition. | Boulder, Colorado: Shambhala, [2026] |
Includes bibliographical references. |
Identifiers: LCCN 2026001219 | ISBN 9781645474906 trade paperback
Subjects: LCSH: Prānāyāma | Hatha yoga
Classification: LCC RA781.7 .R36 2026
LC record available at https://lccn.loc.gov/2026001219

The authorized representative in the EU for product safety and compliance is eucomply OÜ, Pärnu mnt 139b-14, 11317 Tallinn, Estonia, hello@eucompliancepartner.com.

Contents

Preface

In today's popular culture, where Yoga is often reduced to physical posturing, prāṇa to breath, prāṇāyāma to breathing exercises, and Tantra to sensory indulgence, there is a clear need to restore the original, integrative vision of these ancient teachings. This book is written in that spirit—moving against the grain of contemporary reductionism, encouraging an expansive view and profound appreciation of the traditional yogic worldview.

In the yogic tradition, prāṇa is not simply something we respire but a dynamic life principle that animates and moves all things—from breath and food to thought and transcendence. Neither the classical texts nor the living cultural traditions of India view prāṇa as an isolated element; they see it as part of an interconnected web of life. The prāṇa that moves through your breath also stirs oceans, ripens fruits, processes thoughts, circulates in the winds, and sings through birdsongs. It is a living continuum, a subtle thread that weaves together all forms of life. Seen in this way, prāṇa becomes a bridge between the finite and the infinite, nurturing and shaping the body, perception, thought, emotion, speech, and ultimately, spiritual awakening. To reduce it to mere respiratory mechanics is to overlook the profound architecture of reality as articulated in the ancient contemplative traditions of India.

This is not a book about prāṇa as mere breath, nor is it a manual of prāṇāyāma techniques or an attempt to validate yogic wisdom through scientific language. Rather, it invites you to engage with a deeper, more integrative view of prāṇa and to reconsider the way we participate in the world. It invites an inquiry grounded in reverence and wonder, in the spirit of the ancient yogis, where each exploration reveals hidden mysteries and direct experience slowly unfolds into genuine understanding.

This book seeks to renew our appreciation of the yogic worldview by exploring prāṇa across its personal and universal dimensions as experienced in the breath, body, and mind, and reflected in the wider rhythms of nature and cosmic order. Understanding prāṇa as a bridge between the individual and the infinite offers insights that refine not only physical health but also the mental, emotional, social, and spiritual dimensions of life. In this way, prāṇa is no longer merely something we regulate but becomes something we consciously live and embody.

Prāṇa

1

Ancient Yogis and Their Worldview

Prāṇa is everything. I take refuge in Prāṇa.

—Chāndogya Upaniṣad 3.15.4

Imagine standing on the bank of a river. Its waters flow quietly, carrying leaves, light, and whispers from faraway places. You feel its pull, its power, its presence and wonder. *How can I truly know this river? What would it take to understand it?*

One way is to remain on the shore, observing from a distance: collecting water samples, measuring its flow rate and salinity, and analyzing its chemical composition. This method is precise and objective and offers valuable data. But there's another way, and that is to step into the river to feel its current against your body, sense its temperature, taste its waters, and experience its movement with your whole being. This second approach doesn't replace the first; it complements it by offering a direct, experiential understanding. These two modes of knowing reflect what scholars call the *etic* (outsider) and *emic* (insider) perspectives. Both are valuable, each revealing different dimensions of reality.

This book will lean more toward the emic view, seeking to understand prāṇa not merely as an object of study but as a lived and felt phenomenon, much like the ancient yogis did. We are choosing the emic lens—an insider's perspective—for two key reasons:

1. Prāṇa is not an object to be studied from afar, like a mountain or a star. Nor is it reducible to air or oxygen alone. It is a deeply personal experience, felt in our breathing, sensing, feeling, and our very being. We cannot stand apart from it to study it, for it is already an inseparable part of us.

2. Prāṇa is a deeply layered concept, rich in meaning and symbolism, nurtured by the fertile ground of Indian philosophical tradition for thousands of years. Intimately woven into the lived reality of the culture, it has shaped inner life, worldview, and healing traditions across generations. From the insights of the Upaniṣads to temple rituals, from the meditative states of the yogis to the therapeutic wisdom of Āyurveda, prāṇa has remained a

unifying thread—not as an abstract idea, but as a living presence embedded in the cultural memory, language, and personal experience of the land and its people.

Given how deeply prāṇa is rooted in the objective worldview and the subjective consciousness of the culture, we cannot remain on the bank of the river of prāṇa, merely observing from a distance or analyzing isolated samples. To truly grasp its subtle and profound nature, we must step into the river itself—into the perspectives, metaphors, and spiritual pulse of the tradition, immersing ourselves in its language, its logic, and its lived sensibility. Only then can the intuitive depth of prāṇa truly reveal itself, as it did to the ancient yogis.

But who were these ancient seers who explored prāṇa with such an expansive vision? What kind of reality did they perceive? And, perhaps most importantly, can we learn to see as they saw?

THE SIGHT OF THE SEERS, THE ṚṢIS

The oldest reference to prāṇa is found in the Vedas—among the most ancient philosophical and spiritual texts in the world. The Vedic worldview, emerging during the Vedic period (circa 1500 B.C.E. onward), evolving through the Upanishadic era (circa 800 B.C.E. onward), and enriched by later philosophical systems such as Sāṅkhya, Yoga, Vedānta, and Tantra, was grounded in a profound sense of interconnectedness and interdependence. In this vision, life was seen as an intricate web of relationships—with prāṇa flowing as the unifying force through all levels of existence.

The Vedas were not authored in the conventional sense but are said to have been revealed to the ṛṣis—the seers of truth. The ṛṣis were not ordinary thinkers or poets but explorers of extraordinary inner refinement, whose awareness had expanded beyond the conventional limits of sensory perception and intellectual reasoning. Through keen observation of the world around them, sustained self-inquiry, and deep meditation, they explored the profound mysteries of existence. They are called seers not because they merely theorized about reality but because they beheld it directly, perceiving the fundamental unity in all that exists. They birthed a contemplative culture that continues to live even today—one that viewed reality as an interconnected tapestry, where matter, mind, and life were understood as expressions of a single underlying existence (*sat*).

The ṛṣis' intent, inner disposition, and refined powers of perception shaped how the Indic culture expressed the idea of prāṇa across thousands of years. In their holistic vision, carried forward by yogis who followed them, reality was not something to be merely observed or recorded; it was something to be felt, lived, tested, and directly experienced through communion with nature's rhythms and deeper states of awareness.

This vision, summarized as a principle called *piṇḍa brahmāṇḍa siddhānta*, is the understanding that the human being (*piṇḍa*) and the universe (*brahmāṇḍa*) are reflections of each other in both structure and essence. It expresses the simple yet profound idea that the individual and the cosmos are deeply connected as parts of one living whole. Over time, this insight crystallized in the culture as the well-known dictum *Yathā brahmāṇḍe tathā piṇḍe*, or "As in the cosmos, so in the body." This was not merely a poetic metaphor but a lived and observable reality. The ancient seers saw the Sun, Moon, winds, fire, rivers, and seasons not only as external forces but also as energies moving within us, reflected in our breath, thought, digestion, and inner rhythms. This integrative perception, in which the human being is seen as a microcosmic replica of the vast cosmic order, became the foundation for the liberational philosophies of Yoga and the healing modalities of Āyurveda.

Ācārya Caraka, one of the foremost authorities on Āyurveda, emphasized this inseparable connection in his *loka-puruṣa sāmya siddhānta*—the doctrine of sameness between the person and the world (*Caraka Saṃhitā* 5.3–5.4). He affirmed that true health arises when the inner constitution is aligned with the rhythms and laws of the external world, reflecting a state of dynamic equilibrium and holistic well-being. Using this principle, medieval Haṭha Yoga texts like *Siddhasiddhāntapaddhati* (5.1) see the whole cosmos mirrored within the yogi's body.

The ṛṣis' understanding of space and time, too, was far more expansive. They did not view time as a straight line but as a circle, moving through cycles of birth, growth, decay, and renewal. Space, likewise, was not regarded as an empty void but as a conscious field of possibilities. Cosmic phenomena, celestial bodies, and forces of nature were seen as expressions of living deities, archetypes, and intelligences intimately participating in the unfolding of the cosmos.

Their worldview also gave validity to subjective experience, inner perception, and intuitive understanding of subtle realities, not just empirical observation. Existence was not dissected into parts but sensed as a flowing, relational whole. Respiration was not seen as a mere exchange of gases between the lungs and the environment but as an individual's conscious participation in the cosmic dance of life. Meditation and prayer, for them, were not ways of withdrawing from the world but ways of entering into this sacred interconnectedness. The physical and the spiritual were not separate; they were layers of the same lived truth. This way of seeing was so fundamental to their existence that it shaped how they breathed, ate, healed, related, lived, and died.

This vision was not limited to philosophers or sages alone; it infused everyday life and continues to live on in the cultural imagination of the people even today. I remember my father once telling me that he had always wanted to be a professional classical singer but had to give up the dream due to financial hardship, choosing instead to become a lawyer. And yet, he never carried bitterness or regret. Whenever I would ask him if he felt he missed out, he would simply say, "I'll become a singer in my next lifetime." There was genuine hope in his voice, not fantasy. His sense of time was not linear and final but cyclical and expansive, shaped by the vision of the ṛṣis, handed down through generations.

This ideal of time, life, and possibility has quietly shaped how people relate to themselves, to the world around them, and to the deeper currents of their destiny. To uproot lived cultural concepts like prāṇa from the fertile soil of experiential wisdom cultivated over centuries and examine them solely within the narrow petri dish of materialism or modern empiricism is to risk stripping them of their subtlety, depth, nuance, and transformative power.

To truly understand a concept as philosophically rich and existentially impactful as prāṇa, we must honor the perceptual lens of the culture from which it emerged, for it is through this lens that meaning was made and a worldview shaped. Without engaging with this inner logic, we risk diminishing a profound, living reality into a mere intellectual construct.

Our journey, then, is to enter these teachings not just as observers but as humble student-practitioners, willing to stretch the boundaries of our usual ways of thinking and embrace a vision that may feel unfamiliar at first, yet holds the power to illuminate our inner and outer worlds.

OUR VISION AND THE LIMITS OF OUR PERCEPTION

Our worldview depends on the lens through which we view the world. A narrow lens will present a narrow reality, even when we gaze upon vast concepts.

The modern worldview often values analysis over insight and measurement over mystery. In this mindset, prāṇa is generally reduced to breath or oxygen. But when such an approach is applied to subtle, layered, and fundamentally nonmaterial principles like prāṇa, it reaches its natural limit. By focusing solely on what can be observed and measured, we risk overlooking the relational and experiential dimensions of reality. Trying to grasp prāṇa through such a narrow lens is like attempting to appreciate a beautifully prepared meal by analyzing only its calorie content—totally missing the flavor, the feeling, the intention, and the meaning behind the lived experience of eating.

To grasp prāṇa in the yogic sense, we must widen our lens of perception. This entails shifting the very way we relate to reality. Modern methods of inquiry have their place, but they must be complemented with inner awareness, refined intuition, and a recognition of the wholeness that underlies life.

By learning to see through the eyes of the ṛṣis, by opening to their expanded perspective and allowing it to stretch our own limits of knowing, we create the conditions to truly grasp subtle topics like prāṇa. What is required is openness of heart, sensitivity of mind, and depth of perception that allows prāṇa to be appreciated not just as an idea but as a living reality.

YOGA IS THE EXPANSION OF PERCEPTION

At its essence, Yoga is the science of expanding human awareness beyond its habitual limitations. The ancient yogis were not merely concerned with physical fitness or mental relaxation—they aspired to radically deepen human perception to reveal the true nature of reality. Yoga Sūtra 1.2 defines Yoga as *cittavṛtti nirodhaḥ*—the stilling of the mind's fluctuations. Why? Because a restless mind reflects a distorted reality, which in turn gives us suffering. A narrow or agitated mind can only perceive a fragment of the whole, while an expanded, calm mind sees with clarity, depth, and wholeness. When the mind is unburdened through yogic practices, perception becomes more expansive. For example, a person gripped by self-doubt may, through yogic meditation and self-inquiry, begin to witness their thoughts with detachment. In doing so, they may discover a steady state of awareness beneath the turbulence of doubt—one that is content and independent of external validation.

Yoga awakens us from the slumber of mental limitation and reminds us of the vastness of our true nature. This expansion of self-awareness does not come from accumulating more on the outside but from turning inward, shifting from a narrow, material view to a broad, inclusive understanding of ourselves and the world. Yoga is not merely a practice but a lived process grounded in principles born of expanded perception—one that leads us toward inner clarity, freedom, and harmony with life's deeper rhythms. In essence, Yoga is the journey of coming home—from *doing* more to *being* more, from seeking outside to discovering the vastness within.

ENDING INSIGHT

This book invites us to see prāṇa in a broader and more inclusive way—not just as breath but as the living energy that connects and sustains all of existence. Through this expanded understanding, we begin to see how prāṇa flows through every aspect of our existence—body, mind, life, and nature—binding them into a single living reality. As we explore this vision, we will discover how a deeper awareness of prāṇa can transform how we breathe, think, feel, and live, helping us move toward greater harmony with the whole.

Reflection Exercise: Expanding Your Field of Perception

Take a gentle pause to notice the thread that connects everything. Notice how your intention shapes the breath, how your state of mind influences the way you see the world, and how even silence has its own language. As your awareness softens, you may begin to sense not just things but the subtle connections that bring life into harmony.

Now, try doing this in a simple, everyday moment—drinking water, standing in sunlight, eating a piece of fruit, or listening to the breeze. Pause, breathe, and ask yourself the following:

- How does this moment remind me that I'm part of something larger?
- What connects me to it?

Let this quiet contemplation deepen your sense of participation in the larger flow of life. With regular practice, this simple shift in perception can open the doorway to a richer, more connected experience of life.

2

Ideas of Prāṇa Across Yoga Scriptures

From prāṇa all things arise, and into prāṇa they return.

—Chāndogya Upaniṣad 1.11.5

What does the term prāṇa mean? Etymologically, it is derived from *pra* (forward, beginning) and the root *aṇ* (to breathe, to live, to be alive),[1] suggesting the forward movement of life or vital energy—which is an expression of optimal living.

Often translated as "breath" or "life force," prāṇa is the animating principle that sustains life. The *Taittirīya Upaniṣad* (2.3) declares, "Prāṇa is the life span of all beings." Across Indian languages, when someone dies, it is commonly said, "Prāṇa has left their body," reflecting a deep cultural understanding that life and prāṇa are inseparable. In poetic usage, too, one's beloved is often called prāṇa, implying that someone is as essential as life itself. But such definitions and word associations only scratch the surface of the profound idea that is prāṇa.

This is because Sanskrit is a highly contextual language, and in the vast Indic tradition, words like *prāṇa*, *Yoga*, and *Dharma* are considered polysemous, i.e., their meaning shifts and evolves across texts, traditions, contexts, and time periods. Such terms act as semantic bridges, linking the physical, physiological, cosmic, spiritual, and experiential dimensions. Keeping in mind that meaning migrates or morphs across contexts makes us aware of the depth of such concepts and cautions us against reducing them to singular definitions or oversimplifying them. It allows us to respect the richness of the tradition, interpret ideas with sensitivity, and create a thoughtful bridge between ancient wisdom and modern understanding.

While *prāṇa* is commonly translated as "breath," its actual scope in the Vedic tradition stretches far beyond respiration, ranging from "life" to "movement," "vibration," and "awareness" or all of the above.

Let's look at some words that could be considered synonyms of the term *prāṇa*. These are not merely linguistic variations but glimpses into the vastness and subtlety of what prāṇa is. In different contexts, prāṇa is called *vāyu*, the vital wind that governs all movement; *marut*, the divine life force that sustains motion; *vāta*, "that which moves" and regulates activity within the body; and *pavana*, the gentle, flowing breath that purifies and animates life. Thus, prāṇa takes on different names and nuances, each shaped by its philosophical and experiential context.

Such is the importance and glory of prāṇa in the Vedic thought that the *Atharva Veda* (11.4) dedicates an entire hymn of praise to it, called the *Prāṇa Sūkta*. Whether described as breath, air, wind, motion, or *aliveness*, its core meaning remains rooted in the idea of life, motion, and vitality, though the expression varies with the lens through which it is seen.

PRĀṆA—MORE THAN BREATH

In modern Yoga discourse, prāṇa is often equated with physical breath, but while breath is a vital expression of prāṇa, Indic traditions have regarded it as only the most tangible, surface layer of a far deeper, subtler life force.

The *Brahma Sūtra* (2.4.9), a foundational text of Vedānta, states unequivocally that prāṇa is far more than mere physical breath, or respiratory air. The ancient scriptures and scholars affirm that while prāṇa may manifest through breath, it is not limited to it. Rather, it is the deeper animating principle behind breath, life, and awareness itself.

A beautiful verse from the text called *Yogavāsiṣṭha* (6.25.3) presents prāṇa not as a bodily function but as a subtle, self-sustaining force. It is described as constant and ever-moving—the very pulse of life that flows within and beyond us, pervading the greater field of existence. With both material and mental dimensions, prāṇa is said to "stand above," symbolizing its primacy in sustaining life, shaping the mind, and guiding spiritual growth.

Therefore, to understand prāṇa is not to confine it merely to breath or the act of respiration but to begin perceiving it as an unbroken stream of *aliveness*—one that links breath to body, body to mind, mind to life, and life to its infinite source.

THE THREEFOLD FRAMEWORK

The Indian philosophical tradition offers a profound threefold interpretive framework through which any phenomenon, prāṇa included, can be understood. It looks at reality from three complementary perspectives: *ādhidaivika* (the cosmic or divine dimension), *ādhibhautika* (the material or elemental realm), and *ādhyātmika* (the innermost, individual experience). These are not separate or conflicting realities. Instead, they can be equated to the branches, trunk, and roots of a tree, each serving a distinct role, yet inseparably part of one living whole, together offering a complete and integrated vision of life.

The strength of this framework lies in its ability to reveal concepts as a continuum. It allows us to relate to prāṇa not just as breath or biological energy but as part of an interconnected web of cosmic, ecological, and spiritual relationships. It also helps us recognize that prāṇa is not something we merely "possess," but something we *participate in*—a living bridge between body–mind–life. With this foundational understanding in place, we are now ready to explore prāṇa through each of the three dimensions.

THE ĀDHIDAIVIKA VIEW: THE COSMIC DIMENSION

The ādhidaivika dimension is the most expansive and universal perspective, where prāṇa is regarded as the very breath of creation, or Brahman. In this cosmic vision, prāṇa is the source, sustainer, and culmination of all existence, linking the vast universe to the smallest cell through one universal pulse.

Prāṇa is also closely related to the Sun, whose steady light and warmth were seen as the tangible face of the cosmic life force. Thus, in the ādhidaivika understanding, prāṇa spans the entire spectrum from the subtlest stirrings of cosmic intelligence to the blazing brilliance we call the Sun, which sustains all life on Earth.

Prāṇa as Brahman, the Absolute

The *Kauṣītaki Upaniṣad* (2.1) declares, "Prāṇa is Brahman," identifying prāṇa with Absolute Consciousness. This profound insight is echoed in the *Bṛhadāraṇyaka Upaniṣad* (4.4.7), and the *Chāndogya Upaniṣad* (4.10.4), emphasizing prāṇa's ultimate spiritual significance across the Vedic tradition.

Understanding the relationship between Brahman and prāṇa is vital. Brahman is the Absolute Consciousness—pure awareness beyond form or qualities. Yet that same transcendent consciousness expresses itself in a living, tangible way as prāṇa. Prāṇa is Brahman in motion—the presence of the Absolute flowing through creation. It is how the unmanifest becomes manifest, how the unseen becomes felt, and how the infinite becomes intimate. Through prāṇa, the transcendent reveals itself in the living world.

When we look closely at the world around us, one truth stands out: everything is in motion. From the blink of an eye to the orbit of planets and the swirl of atoms, everything in the universe expresses itself through movement. But what animates this ceaseless dance? The ancient yogis, through deep meditative insight, perceived a subtle, all-pervading presence underlying every act of motion and manifestation—prāṇa.

In recognition of prāṇa's supreme role, the *Bṛhadāraṇyaka Upaniṣad* (6.1.1) and the *Chāndogya Upaniṣad* (5.1.1) both declare it the oldest and the greatest—the original, primal force from which everything arises and is sustained.

This is also why the *Ṛg Veda* (10.168.3) calls prāṇa the firstborn. It was the cosmic ignition, the universe's own moment of awakening, the "bang" in the big bang, so to speak—propelling energy, matter, and consciousness into their boundless journey. Prāṇa is thus the "breath" of creation, the unseen current that enlivens and connects the cosmos and its creation.

Since Brahman is consciousness itself, all that emerges from it carries consciousness, too—sometimes fully awake, sometimes latent—expressed in infinite gradations from the inertia of a stone to the awakened awareness of a sage. This is the universe that the ṛṣis and yogis have perceived in their evolved meditative states—a universe that is not inert matter but a vast, interconnected field of *aliveness*. The *Chāndogya Upaniṣad* (7.15.1) gives an apt metaphor for this, saying "Just as the spokes of a wheel are fastened to the hub, so is everything fastened to prāṇa." Far beyond a functional term like *energy* or *force*, prāṇa is the very pulse of existence, the animating essence of all life and motion across the universe.

Prāṇa as the Sun

We now turn to a more visible cosmic expression of prāṇa—the Sun. In the Vedic vision, the Sun is the grandest embodiment of prāṇa, ever-present, life-giving, and unwavering. In an age without artificial light, heat, or electricity, the Sun was, for the ancient yogis, far more than a celestial body. It was a living presence, a constant source of energy and assurance. Naturally, it came to represent the origin of all vitality, movement, and transformation. Its steady light and warmth were seen as the tangible face of the cosmic life force. As the *Praśna Upaniṣad* (1.5 and 3.8) affirms, "The Sun indeed is the prāṇa," and elsewhere (1.8) declares it *prāṇaḥ prajānām*, "the life of all beings." The Sun's constancy made it the visible face of the invisible life force.

While the Sun is the most visible expression of cosmic prāṇa, it is not the only source through which we can feel its presence. Sometimes simply reflecting on what we are made of can awaken a deep sense of wonder. Just imagine—the hydrogen in your body was formed within moments of the big bang, more than thirteen billion years ago. The oxygen you breathe was born in the hearts of ancient stars, scattered across galaxies, and later shaped by Earth's oceans and living organisms into the element that sustains your life today. Every particle in you has traveled through stars, oceans, forests, and countless living beings before arriving here, now, as you.

You are not separate from the universe; you are its *continuation*, its living expression. The same life force that first set matter into motion still flows through stars, trees, rivers, and your own heartbeat. It has never stopped. To be alive is to participate in this timeless current of prāṇa—the pulse of existence moving through all that is.

This interconnected flow of life is what brings us to the ādhibhautika dimension of prāṇa—the prāṇa expressed through the natural world and all its living forms.

THE ĀDHIBHAUTIKA DIMENSION: THE LIVING BREATH OF THE WORLD AROUND US

The natural drive toward life, the instinct to survive and continue, is a clear sign of prāṇa at work. It enlivens, connects, and sustains all forms of life on Earth. Just as the Sun is a radiant expression of prāṇa, so too are the five elements—earth, water, fire, air, and space—and each is infused with its presence. Prāṇa is what gives the elements their movement and vitality and nurtures the living essence within nature in countless ways. It flows in the rushing rivers, rises with the sap in plants, radiates through sunlight, and hums in the wind that carries seeds across fields. It stirs in the buzzing of bees, the blooming of flowers, the cycles of the Moon, and the gentle warmth of the soil that nourishes roots. Prāṇa is the quiet intelligence behind the changing seasons, the migration of birds, and the harmony of biological ecosystems. It sustains not just individual life-forms but the entire rhythm and balance of the natural world. Prāṇa sustains the life and growth of all vegetation and thus nourishes the earth. The *Praśna Upaniṣad* (2.10), declares, "O Prāṇa, when you pour down as rain, then your creatures continue to be in a happy mood under the belief, 'Food will be produced to our hearts' content.'"[2]

It is through prāṇa's motile force that the plants absorb sunlight, draw water and nutrients from the soil, and respond to their environment. The blooming of flowers, the turning of leaves toward the Sun, the emergence of roots—all are signs of prāṇa at work. Though plants may not have a nervous system like animals, their *aliveness* is undeniable, and it is through the flow of prāṇa that they maintain their growth, healing, and reproduction.

Through the prāṇic lens, plants are not seen as passive products of nature but living beings pulsing with the subtle life essence. This life essence flows through the interconnected web of life. As animals graze on the nourished plants, they absorb this vitality, carrying it into their own bodies and life processes. When humans consume plants, especially those that are fresh, vibrant, and close to nature, we too draw in the prāṇa embedded within them. This energy transfer not only nourishes our physical tissues but also supports our mental clarity, emotional balance, and spiritual receptivity.

The *Chāndogya Upaniṣad* (6.6.3) says that prāṇa is the subtlest essence of water. When we drink water, we absorb the *jīvana tattva*—the life essence—contained in it. This is why in Sanskrit, *jala* (water) is also referred to as *jīvana* (life). Water is not seen merely as a specific combination of hydrogen and oxygen molecules but as the carrier of prāṇa, the very essence that sustains life. Rivers are seen as living expressions of prāṇa, sustaining ecosystems, nourishing civilizations, and bringing life wherever they flow. In deep recognition of this truth, Indian culture reveres rivers as mothers and deities, such as Mother Gaṅgā, honoring not just their physical presence but the sacred prāṇic essence in their flow—the very pulse of life that has nourished generations.

In many indigenous traditions of India, trees, too, are revered as sacred carriers of prāṇa. They are cherished like family and celebrated during festivals—an offering of heartfelt gratitude for the life and nourishment they provide. This reverence evokes a natural ethic of conservation, where devotion becomes protection. Trees like the peepal (*Ficus religiosa*), banyan (*Ficus benghalensis*), and neem (*Azadirachta indica*) are not only vital to the environment but are also elevated to the status of deities, woven into the cultural and spiritual life of the people.

The life-giving essence of prāṇa flows in a continuous cycle—from soil to seed, plant to animal, and animal to human—forming an unbroken current of living energy.

The *Prāṇa Sūkta* (a hymn in the *Atharva Veda* 11.4.10) uses the metaphor of a father caring for his son to express how prāṇa nurtures and protects all creatures.

Thus, prāṇa is not seen as a static force but a dynamic stream that connects all beings in a shared field of vitality, sustaining and renewing life across forms and species. It is this prāṇa flow that powers the food chain, nourishing everything on the planet from the tiniest bacteria to the mightiest elephant.

When we begin to see prāṇa as the subtle current uniting soil, water, plants, animals, and humans, ecological awareness stops being an abstract idea and becomes a deeply personal relationship. If we felt every tree we cut, every river we pollute, and every patch of earth we drain of life as a disturbance in the shared breath of life, would we act differently? Could reverence for prāṇa inspire us to protect the delicate weave of interdependence that sustains us all? In remembering this truth, we find hope that by honoring prāṇa, we can restore balance, vitality, and harmony to the living world.

THE ĀDHYĀTMIKA VIEW: THE PERSONAL DIMENSION OF PRĀṆA

The ādhyātmika view refers to the innermost or subjective dimension of reality. Just as prāṇa permeates every aspect of the universe, so, too, does it permeate every aspect of the human person: physical, physiological, psychological, and even social.

In *Praśna Upaniṣad* (3.1–3.3), it is asked, "From where is this prāṇa born?" The teacher responds with a profound truth: "From the Self, indeed, this prāṇa is born." This reminds us that at the individualized, personal level, prāṇa is an extension of the True Self.

In Sanskrit, and many other Indian languages, a sentient being is called *prāṇi*, the one who lives through prāṇa. To be a prāṇi is to be a living expression of prāṇa. The very structure of the word reflects an intuitive truth deeply rooted in the Indic worldview: life, awareness, and vitality are inseparable from the presence of prāṇa.

Prāṇa plays a defining role in the existence and the duration of the individual physical self. The universal prāṇa, in itself, is beyond time—for past, future, and all of existence are established within it. Yet, at the individual level, prāṇa determines the very span of life for all beings (*Taittirīya Upaniṣad* 2.3.1). Its entry into the body animates the physical form, and its withdrawal dissolves that individuality back into the whole. When prāṇa leaves, the body ceases to live; hence, the *Atharva Veda* (11.4.11) addresses prāṇa as *mṛtyu*, death itself.

A verse from the *Śatapatha Brāhmaṇa* (10.3.3.6) says that in the stillness of sleep, when all outward faculties rest, the senses and the mind withdraw into prāṇa and from prāṇa, they arise again upon waking. This suggests that prāṇa is the very inner hub of awareness, the silent axis around which all the activities of the mind and senses turn, organizing and harmonizing our entire experience of life as an individual.

The Indic philosophical tradition offers multiple models to describe the human person. Every model integrates multiple dimensions of human existence—physical, prāṇic, mental, and spiritual—reflecting a holistic and layered understanding of the self.

The *pañcakośa* model, from the *Taittirīya Upaniṣad* (3.1–6), describes the human being as consisting of five concentric layers or sheaths, from the gross physical to the subtlest spiritual, each one enveloping the other. This model places prāṇa as the vital sheath (*prāṇamaya kośa*) that connects the physical body (*annamaya kośa*) with the mind (*manomaya kośa*), acting as the bridge between gross matter and the subtle mind.

Tantric traditions, too, present a dynamic vision of the human being composed of a subtle energy body threaded with *nāḍīs* (energy channels), spinning cakras (energy centers), and a dormant potential known as kuṇḍalinī. Prāṇa flows through the nāḍīs, governing not just physiological functions but also the emotional, mental, and spiritual states.

Āyurveda echoes this integrated view, identifying prāṇa vāyu as critical for vitality, motion, and nurturing of the body–mind system—including respiration, sensory perception, and mental clarity. Any imbalance or obstruction in the flow of prāṇa is said to result in systemic disharmony or disease. The key to health and well-being is to maintain harmony of prāṇa. Ācārya Caraka, in *Caraka Saṃhitā, Sūtra Sthāna* (chapter 12), says, "Prāṇa (vāyu) is the initiator of all kinds of activities within the body, the controller and impellor of all mental functions, and the employer of all sensory faculties."

This is how all systems of Indic thought integrate prāṇa into their framework of the human being, revealing not only its central role but also the depth and breadth of its influence across every layer of human existence. Such integration points to the comprehensive impact of prāṇa on the individual, from bodily health to mental clarity and spiritual awakening.

Prāṇa as Breath

There is a story in the *Chāndogya Upaniṣad* (5.1.6–15) that beautifully illustrates the supremacy of prāṇa among all faculties of the body. In a simple yet profound way, it shows how it is not just another function alongside speech, sight, or thought but the very force that holds them all together and gives them life.

Once, the organs—speech, eyes, ears, mind, and prāṇa—began to quarrel among themselves, each claiming to be the most important and supreme. To settle the debate, they decided that one by one, each would withdraw from the body to see what would happen. First, speech left, and though the body became mute, it still lived. Then the eyes left, and though the body became blind, it continued to survive. Next, the ears departed; the body became deaf but remained alive. Even the mind withdrew, and though confused and forgetful, the body still functioned.

Finally, when prāṇa began to leave, all the other organs panicked. They rushed to prāṇa and pleaded for it to stay, realizing that without it, none of them could function and the body itself would perish. The story ends with all the organs accepting that prāṇa is indeed the supreme among them; it is the sustaining force holding all faculties together. From that ancient story, we are reminded that it is the breath—the movement of prāṇa—that truly animates the body and turns mere structure into living presence.

The Body of Breath

Breath is what turns the body from structure into *aliveness*—animating flesh, awakening rhythm, and keeping every cell in motion. With every inhale, the chest widens, the ribs lift, and the diaphragm moves down to make space for air to fill the lungs. As the diaphragm descends, it gently massages the abdominal organs, promoting subtle movement within the digestive tract and improving circulation. This internal, wave-like action also helps stabilize the spine, creating a foundational anchor from which all other movement in the body initiates. A fully connected breath is a full-body movement. The rhythmic movement of the diaphragm also supports the body's cleansing systems, aiding lymphatic flow and assisting in the purification of blood.

This physical rhythm naturally merges into a deeper physiological intelligence. With each breath, oxygen enters the bloodstream and begins its journey to every cell, sustaining renewal and vitality. Every exhale carries the quiet wisdom of gas exchange—the body's innate knowing of what to keep and what to release—maintaining a delicate balance essential to life. This simple, steady rhythm continues without our command, yet it is also the most direct way to return to ourselves.

When we pause to truly feel the breath, we sense how intimately it shapes both body and brain: shallow breaths tighten the chest and quicken the pulse, while deeper ones soften the muscles, calm the heart, and steady the thoughts. The breath reflects emotions. The brain, as an electrochemical organ, moves in resonance with the rhythm of breathing—every inhale subtly excites neural activity, while every exhale encourages calm and regulation through the parasympathetic system. Slow, steady breathing balances this dance, synchronizing heart rhythms and brain waves, allowing clarity and ease to emerge. Each breath reminds us that life moves through this body in a living rhythm and that by embodying this flow consciously, we learn what it means to truly dwell in our own physical being. Yet, the breath does more than sustain the body; it also shapes the inner world of our thoughts, emotions, and awareness.

The relationship between prāṇa as breath and the mind is so deep and intricate that it deserves to be treated as a chapter in its own right. Prāṇa's influence as breath on thought, emotion, attention, and inner stillness lies at the heart of Yoga psychology. We will explore this vital connection in depth in the next chapter.

ENDING INSIGHT

Through the threefold lens of ādhidaivika (cosmic), ādhibhautika (natural), and ādhyātmika (individual), we see prāṇa not as three realities but as one living presence viewed from different angles. Just as rain, rivers, and drinking water are forms of the same element, the prāṇa within us is continuous with that which moves stars, winds, and cells. It is the thread weaving the universe, nature, and self into one seamless whole.

So, if you ever feel small, lonely, or not good enough, remember this: The universe didn't just create you; it continues to live through you. You are not separate from the cosmic rhythm; you are its intimate expression. To bask in sunlight, drink water, eat, move, speak, or simply sit in stillness is to participate in the timeless dance of existence, where nothing is ordinary and everything pulses with life. In every moment, prāṇa moves through you, not as something that you have, but as the very force that you *are*.

Awakening the Breath of Life: The Three Ws Practice

One simple way to embody the holistic vision of prāṇa in our daily life is to cultivate what I call the three *ws*: wonderment, watchfulness, and warmth.

1. **Wonderment at the cosmos (ādhidaivika prāṇa)** invites us to look beyond our small concerns and open to the immensity of existence. The stars, the seasons, the unseen forces moving the universe—all breathe with us. When we cultivate awe for the cosmic prāṇa, we remember that each breath is shared with the same life force that spins the galaxies. This sense of wonder expands our vision and lifts our spirit.

2. **Watchfulness over nature (ādhibhautika prāṇa)** grounds this cosmic vision in care for the living world. The rivers, forests, winds, and soil carry the same prāṇa that sustains our bodies. To protect and preserve them is to honor our own life force. Watchfulness here means active stewardship—living with consideration, consuming mindfully, and restoring balance wherever we can.

3. **Warmth toward ourselves (ādhyātmika prāṇa)** brings prāṇa into the most intimate sphere—our own inner life. It begins with the quiet art of treating ourselves with gentleness, living with moderation, regulating our thoughts, and walking the path of yogic self-transformation with patience. When we listen to our needs and hold space for our emotions without judgment, we nourish our breath with kindness, creating an inner reservoir of steadiness and compassion. From this wellspring, our warmth naturally flows outward—touching our relationships, our community, and every life we encounter.

To integrate wonderment, watchfulness, and warmth is to live in recognition that we are participating in the vast and sacred web of life—feeling its flow in the cosmos, in nature, and within our own being. When we consciously attune to these dimensions, breathing ceases to be a mere bodily act and becomes a dynamic bridge linking the infinite expanse and the intimate self.

In this way, prāṇa is not an abstract concept but the very ground of our wholeness, where every breath becomes a gentle reminder, inviting us to return to balance, to move with purpose, to dwell in presence, and to softly ask, *What might unfold if I truly remembered how limitless I really am?*

3

Prāṇa as Breath and Mind

The mind is tied to prāṇa.

—Chāndogya Upaniṣad 6.8.2

In some yogic texts, the mind is compared to a mirror that reflects both the self and the world. When this mirror becomes clouded, our perception gets distorted, and we experience suffering. A small mark on the mirror may seem like a flaw in ourselves—for example, even a casual comment can hurt us deeply when our sense of self is already fragile. Recognizing the importance of the mind, the *Amṛtabindu Upaniṣad* (2) asserts, "The mind alone is the cause of bondage and liberation."

This is why the working goal of Yoga is *chitta-śuddhi* (cleansing of the mind). It is also why Yoga Sūtra 1.2 declares, *Yogaś citta-vṛtti-nirodhaḥ* (Yoga is the stilling of the mind's fluctuations), implying that clarity of mind is essential for realizing one's own true nature. A refined mind mirrors the self and the world without distortion. This is precisely where Yoga's understanding of prāṇa as breath and its link to the mind becomes vital.

PRĀṆA, MIND, AND PUPPETS OF PATTERNS

What is truly remarkable is how the ancient yogis delved deeply into the intricate relationship between prāṇa and the mind through direct observation and meditation. They did not view breath merely as a physical process but also as a psychological reality—a gateway to the subtle realms of the mind.

The profound complementariness between prāṇa and mind is captured beautifully via analogies across yogic literature. For example, according to the *Yogavāsiṣṭha* (5.91.14–16), the mind grows like a tree from two seeds: the vibration of prāṇa and the force of deep-rooted patterns. When prāṇa vibrations flow through the network of nāḍīs, they activate mental awareness (*saṃvedanā*). When this flow stops, mental activity also comes to a standstill. What we call "the world" is actually a projection created by the vibrations of prāṇa, seen through the filter of the mind—just as a movie appears real when light flickers through a film reel.

These prāṇa vibrations stir the mind, keep the sense faculties active, create perception, and drive the unfolding of our joys and sorrows. But when the vibrations of prāṇa slow down, the movements of the mind also become calm and are no longer pushed or pulled by old patterns. This is real *śānti*, or inner peace. Without inner peace, the mind and body, moved by prāṇa, are like puppets pulled by invisible strings—the dancing puppets of mental patterns in life's drama. The process of Yoga restores our ability to move freely with conscious choice rather than being hijacked by forces of seeded patterns (*saṃskāra*).

Such analogies reflect not mere poetic creativity but precise insight into the intimate relationship between prāṇa and mind. These insights, refined through generations of inner exploration, reveal that the two are not separate forces but complementary aspects of one integrated system—two sides of the same coin. Prāṇa is the energetic dimension, and mind is the cognitive—each sustaining the other's function, like electricity and a computer program. Here, prāṇa is the current that enables processing, and mind is the code that shapes that energy into thought, perception, and action.

From the perspective of the ancient yogis, to be truly alive is not merely to breathe but to recognize and attune ourselves to the vibratory intelligence of prāṇa that silently orchestrates the functions of body and mind. Our experience of life is continually shaped by the breath we take and the mind through which we perceive life. This profound interplay between prāṇa and mind is not metaphorical; it is a foundational principle of yogic psychology and the heart of its transformative practice.

Prāṇa as Breath and Mind Regulation

The most tangible expression of the vibratory prāṇa that animates the body and the mind is the respiratory breath—*śvāsa-praśvāsa*, the rhythm of inhalation and exhalation. The physical breath is not just an exchange of gases but a wave in the deeper ocean of prāṇic vibration. Just as brain waves reflect inner mental states and their outer expression, our breath waves modulate our mental workings and external behavior.

The Haṭha yogis knew this correlation very well. The *Haṭha Yoga Pradīpikā* (2.2) declares, "When the breath moves, the mind moves; when the breath is still, the mind becomes still."

You may have noticed this yourself—how a tense conversation, a sudden worry, or even excitement changes your breathing without you realizing it. The breath becomes shallow, rapid, or uneven. But when you pause and take a few deep, mindful breaths, something shifts—the mind begins to settle, and a quiet space opens within. This is because the breath serves as the bridge between body and mind. By refining our breathing pattern through awareness and regulation, we learn to fine-tune the subtle workings of the mind.

Conscious regulation of the breath is known as prāṇāyāma. For the ancient yogis, prāṇāyāma was far more than a respiratory exercise; it was a powerful method of inner purification and transformation. It served as a bridge to deeper meditative absorption (samādhi), where ingrained patterns (saṃskāras) could be dissolved, revealing the self in its purest form. By working on the breath, one can gradually filter out the silt of limiting conditioning accumulated over lifetimes, allowing the pond of the mind to regain its original clarity and stillness. In this purified stillness, the depth of True Self becomes visible.

The *Kauṣītaki Upaniṣad* (2.1) expresses this relationship beautifully, stating that the mind is the messenger of prāṇa, acting as the link between the outer world and the inner world. Just as a messenger carries information from one place to another, the mind carries information from the outer world into the inner field of prāṇa vibrations where it is received, perceived, and experienced.

In the pañcakośa model, the prāṇamaya kośa—the prāṇa layer—stands between the physical and mental layers, animating the body and senses on one side while influencing thought and emotion on the other. Its central placement between the annamaya kośa and manomaya kośa reflects the experiential truth that our breath energy continually shapes our mental state. The bridge-like role of the prāṇamaya kośa affirms what ancient yogis knew intuitively: To access the mind, access prāṇa. The *Yogaśikhā Upaniṣad* (60) clearly declares, "There is no means of controlling the mind other than the regulation of prāṇa."

This understanding has profound therapeutic implications: A person experiencing anxiety may find it difficult to directly calm the agitated mind, yet when approached through gentle regulation of the breath, or specific forms of prāṇāyāma, the same mind begins to shift subtly, opening itself to balance and healing.

Similar to the pañcakośa model, the Yoga Sūtras too give us a distilled science of mental regulation. They recognize the vital role of breath management in calming the mind. Yoga Sūtra 1.34 states, "Through exhalation and retention of breath, [the mind becomes quiet]." Here, Maharṣi Patañjali implies that the rhythm and quality of breath regulate the mental workings, and one's control over prāṇa is a gateway to accessing subtler states of mind. In other words, breath is not just a support for meditation; it is a profound instrument of mental transformation.

When the breath is made steady, the mind too becomes steady, allowing us to respond to life with greater presence and less reactivity. By consciously realigning the breath, we can interrupt the loop of impulsive reactions that create suffering in our lives. Imagine—the key to calming the mind has been right under our nose all along, quite literally in the breath. Each inhale and exhale becomes a gentle reminder that the power to restore balance, focus, and peace has always been within us.

The insight that breath modulation shapes mental and emotional health is not limited to ancient texts; it is increasingly confirmed by clinical research and modern therapeutic models.[3]

Prāṇa as Communication

While we have seen how prāṇa is intimately connected to the mind, its role is not confined to inner workings alone; it also governs how we express, especially through speech (*vāc*).

In yogic thought, breath and speech are considered inseparable companions. Communication via language is nothing but the modulation of sound through controlled movement of breath.

The *Kauṣītaki Upaniṣad* (2.5) observes that a person offers their breath into speech, and their speech back into breath—revealing their intimate unity. You can feel this truth in your own experience. Notice how your voice trembles when you're anxious, rises when you're angry, or softens when you feel calm and open. The rhythm and tone of your speech follow the rhythm of your breath. When the breath is steady, words flow with ease and clarity; when it is restless, speech carries tension. Our voice, in that sense, is a mirror of our inner state—every word we speak carries the signature of our breath.

This is why Sanskrit linguistics classifies letters into *mahāprāṇa* (aspirated, "great breath") and *alpaprāṇa* (unaspirated, "lesser breath"), which reflects how breath awareness is embedded in the very construction of Sanskrit language. Moreover, in Vedic chanting, modulation of breath becomes crucial and sacred through specific rules like *swara* (intonation—the smooth, even tone of inhalation and exhalation), *balam* (strength—the balanced effort and steadiness with which the breath moves), and *mātrā* (duration—the measured rhythm and timing of each breath), showing how prāṇa is harnessed not just for verbal expression but also for sacred transmission.

In Indic culture, symbolism runs deep. The goddess Sarasvatī, revered as Vāc Devī—the goddess of speech—is depicted riding a swan (*haṃsa*), a symbol of the subtle, serene breath. Think of how a swan glides effortlessly over still waters—calm, graceful, and unhurried. In the same way, when our breath flows quietly and evenly, the mind too becomes tranquil and steady beneath the surface. The imagery of Sarasvatī on the *haṃsa* reminds us that when breath moves in calm harmony, words become a reflection of inner wisdom.

The *Śatapatha Brāhmaṇa* (10.1.1.9), too, expresses this dynamic relationship: "Prāṇa is the husband, speech is the wife—together they are a couple." This metaphor reflects the intimate union of breath and speech, where breath is the energy and speech its expression. Just as a couple together gives rise to new life, so, too, does the union of breath and speech gives rise to language and meaning.

Interestingly, even in silence, our breath continues to communicate. Think about it: When someone sighs heavily or breathes in short, sharp bursts, we instantly sense their fatigue or frustration. And when another person breathes slowly and evenly, don't they seem calm, grounded, and at ease? Experienced Yoga teachers often read a student's breath this way while teaching a class, listening to what words cannot convey. The truth is, breath is its own language—the quiet communicator of our inner world.

Breath is also a language through which the body communicates with itself. Each breath causes physical movement that sends a stream of neural signals from the lungs to the brain, especially via the vagus nerve and interoceptive pathways, informing the brain about the internal state of the body. These messages help regulate homeostasis, influence autonomic nervous system balance, and even shape emotional tone and cognitive clarity. This bidirectional loop of communication between breath and brain ensures that physiological responses such as heart rate, digestion, and hormonal secretions are constantly adjusted to match the needs of the moment. In essence, breath is the body's internal language, translating signals into coordinated physiological action.

Furthermore, the rhythm and depth of breathing directly affect the level of gases in the blood, which in turn modulates blood pH, vascular tone, and nervous system balance. Slow, diaphragmatic breathing promotes optimal gas exchange, helping maintain a healthy CO_2 level, which is essential for proper oxygen delivery to tissues—a phenomenon known as the Bohr effect.[4] On the other hand, rapid or shallow breathing often leads to hypocapnia (low CO_2), which can cause blood vessels to constrict, reducing blood flow to the brain and increasing anxiety, dizziness, and even cognitive fog.[5]

What this really shows is that every breath is like a live conversation happening inside us between body, brain, and mind. Each inhale and exhale sends signals that regulate our chemistry, emotions, and energy levels. In this way, breath becomes the body's built-in communication system, coordinating our physical, physiological, and psychological states moment by moment. Thus, breath truly is the "language" the body speaks—with itself and with the world.

Prāṇa as Neural Vibrations

Yoga texts like the *Yogavāsiṣṭha* (5.91.17–18) talk about the vibrational nature of prāṇa, called *prāṇa-spandana*. The term *spandana* means "vibration," "oscillation," or "pulse," and prāṇa-spandana is the vibrational energy (*spandana shakti*) that enables the mind to function.

Prāṇa-spandana has parallels in modern neurophysiology. Our sensory and cognitive functions depend on the firing of neural networks made possible by membrane potential, the fundamental bioelectrical polarity that enables neurons to generate impulses.[6] Thought, perception, and states of mind arise from these electrochemical signals, where tiny voltage shifts move across neural pathways. These signals manifest as measurable brain waves, which are rhythmic oscillations remarkably similar to the yogic notion of spandana. Brain waves could be seen as modern analogues of prāṇic vibrations, expressing various states of consciousness such as wakefulness, dreaming, or deep meditation.

Breath plays a central role in modulating these energetic oscillations. Breath rhythm influences heart rate variability, which in turn entrains brain wave activity and emotional regulation.[7] This process strongly reflects the yogic insight that prāṇa vibrations govern the mind.

In this way, the concept of prāṇa-spandana, or prāṇic vibrations, acts as a bridge between the ancient yogic understanding of life energy and the scientific view of the nervous system as an electrical and vibrational information network.

In the end, the difference between modern and yogic views may lie less in their principles and more in their language. At the physiological level, what Yoga describes as prāṇa, modern science describes as neural or electrical activity—two ways of speaking about the same living rhythm. What the ancient yogis sensed as spandana (vibration or pulse), science measures as oscillation, voltage, or frequency. Both point to a rhythmic intelligence that animates body and mind alike. Learning to bridge these two languages may help us develop a more complete understanding of Yoga, health, healing, and consciousness.

PRĀṆA AND ENERGETIC BLOCKAGES

Emotions, traumas, and memories are increasingly understood to have bodily expressions—showing up as chronic muscle tension, imbalanced posture, or irregular breathing patterns. We've all felt it: shoulders tightening with stress, the chest constricting with worry, or the breath turning shallow when we're anxious. Over time, these patterns can disrupt the body–mind harmony, leaving us feeling unsettled, tired, or emotionally heavy.

In yogic understanding, such restrictions are known as

granthis—energetic knots or blockages where the natural flow of prāṇa becomes constricted or held. Sri Kṣemarāja in the *Netratantra* (7.1) says that granthis are formed when consciousness or intelligent awareness moving through the nāḍīs is blocked. The *Svacchandatantra* (4.364) describes granthis as places where prāṇa energy (*prāṇaśakti*) deteriorates due to distortion in its flow. Thus, when the flow of prāṇa is obstructed, the body–mind system loses coherence, leading to dysfunction in both subtle and gross physiology. Over time, such blockages can disrupt the body's natural harmony, leading to body–mind imbalances. The yogis state that the knots need to be pierced (*bheda*) through prāṇic practices and meditation to liberate one's awareness.

In a specific yogic modality called *prāṇa dhāraṇā*, prāṇa is consciously redirected to dissolve the granthis and restore integration between body and mind. Breath becomes the natural way to release energetic blockages. When one breathes consciously, with intention and attention, prāṇa begins to move in areas where it was previously stuck. This leads to a gradual softening of old blockages and resistances to create conditions for emotional healing. For example, consider someone who has experienced an emotional trauma such as the sudden loss of a loved one and over time begins to feel tightness or constriction in their chest along with shallow breathing. Despite an intellectual understanding that one needs to move on, the grief feels stuck in the body. When this person begins a conscious breathing or prāṇāyāma practice—say, gentle deep breathing with focused awareness—they may initially encounter discomfort or emotional waves. But over time, breath begins to reach those frozen areas in the chest. With each session, the breath softens the inner contraction, and tears may arise not from sadness alone but as a physiological release of stored emotion. Gradually, the feeling of being stuck begins to ease. The gentle, unforced breath brings life back to those frozen areas, becoming the channel through which prāṇic intelligence reconnects mind and body, restoring calm, wholeness, and vitality.

From the scientific perspective, this happens because slow, conscious breathing activates the parasympathetic nervous system, particularly the vagus nerve, reducing sympathetic overdrive (fight or flight) and enhancing emotional regulation through improved heart rate variability and limbic system balance. Over time, this shift generates neuroplasticity and helps rewire trauma-conditioned neural pathways, allowing stored emotional energy to be released safely.

Modern tools like biofeedback and heart-rate variability trackers also confirm that mindful breathing can calm the mind and balance the body. These tools show that slow, deep breathing helps relax the nervous system, quiet emotional reactivity, and bring the body and mind into greater harmony. In this way, the breath becomes a gentle but powerful tool for restoring balance and emotional stability.

Working with prāṇa is a gateway to mental transformation—not symbolically but biologically and experientially.

PRĀṆA LEAKAGE, PACE OF BREATH, AND SPAN OF LIFE

In today's world, many of us feel chronically drained—an experience that can be understood as prāṇa leakage, a gradual loss of vital energy due to overstimulation. Think about it: How often do we reach for our phone the moment there's silence or scroll endlessly only to feel more tired? Sensory overload from screens, noise, and busyness overwhelms the brain's filters, triggering stress responses and deep fatigue. In yogic terms, this constant overactivation disperses prāṇa through erratic breathing, racing heartbeat, and scattered focus, leaving us reactive instead of centered. The U.S. Department of Health and Human Services notes a clear link between excessive screen time and increased anxiety and depressive symptoms in adolescents.[8]

The Yoga tradition has always connected loss of vitality to the rate of breath. The *Ṛg Veda* (1.66.1) equates prāṇa to lifespan, thus also equating loss of prāṇa to loss of life. Ancient seers observed that animals with slower, deeper breathing, like tortoises and elephants, tend to live longer, whereas those with rapid, shallow breathing, like rabbits or dogs, often have short lifespans. From this, they inferred that to rush through the breaths is quite literally to shorten one's life. Modern physiology reflects this insight: Consistently high respiratory rates increase metabolic demand, oxidative stress, and systemic inflammation, contributing to cellular aging and reduced longevity.[9] In this light, the popular saying "Live fast, die young" becomes physiologically accurate—rapid breathing and overstimulation exhaust prāṇa at an accelerated pace. By consciously slowing down the breath rate and practicing sensory regulation we can conserve prāṇa, restore balance to the nervous system, and create conditions for a longer, steadier, and more vibrant life. Maybe living well was never about doing more but about breathing less—and feeling more. The next time life feels like it's moving too fast, perhaps all it's asking is for you to slow your breathing.

ENDING INSIGHT

In the chapters we have explored so far, prāṇa emerges as a multidimensional reality expressing itself across three levels: ādhidaivika (cosmic/divine), ādhibhautika (natural/elemental), and ādhyātmika (individual/spiritual). In the broadest sense, prāṇa's core characteristics can be summarized as follows:

1. **Conscious intelligence** (*caitanya-śakti*): Prāṇa is the light of consciousness (Brahman's creative energy) that infuses life with the capacity for intelligence, order, and vitality.

2. **Movement** (*gati*): Prāṇa is the unseen principle of motion that animates all activity, from the breath and blood flow to the movement of thought and the expansion of the cosmos.

3. **Connector of dimensions** (*setu*): Prāṇa acts as the common, living thread that flows from the Absolute into the individual, sustaining and regulating all vital systems.

All the qualities of prāṇa find a living expression in the form of the Hindu deity Hanumān. In the epics, he stands as the very embodiment of life's vital force—dynamic, intelligent, and devoted. Born as Vāyu Putra, the "son of the wind god, Vāyu," Hanumān mirrors the boundless, tireless movement of prāṇa itself. His great leap across the ocean to reach Sītā and be the link between her and Rāma, and his zest in carrying the mountain of healing herbs to revive Lakṣmaṇa, symbolize how prāṇa moves, links, and sustains life. Yet beyond his strength, Hanumān's true power lies in his devotion to Rāma, the embodiment of Absolute Consciousness (Brahman). In offering each breath in service to Rāma, Hanumān reminds us that prāṇa is not ours to possess. It is the Divine Consciousness moving through all creation. For centuries, Yoga practitioners have contemplated Hanumān, both as deity and symbol, as a reminder that every breath is a sacred, intelligent force meant to uphold awareness, evoke purposeful enthusiasm, and carry us toward the highest goal of life: self-realization.

When prāṇa is understood in this way, its characteristics dissolve the sense of fragmentation in life. We realize that the same force that moves the stars nourishes our body and flows gently through our breath. Relating to prāṇa in this way brings balance, clarity, and vitality while deepening our reverence for all forms of life.

Breath Exploration Exercise: Deep, Slow Breath

This simple yet foundational practice, called *dīrgha śvāsa*, gently lengthens and deepens the natural breath to calm the mind, revealing, through direct experience, how breath and mental state mirror each other.

Instructions

1. Sit comfortably with a straight spine. Soften the shoulders and jaw. Close the eyes.

2. Take three gentle, natural breaths—don't modulate, just notice and allow yourself to become aware of your breath.

3. Now, inhale slowly through the nose for a comfortable count of say 4. Sense the breath filling the lower belly, then the ribs, then the chest—a gentle, smooth expansion.

4. Exhale slowly through the nose for a slightly longer comfortable count of 5 or 6.* Let the chest sink, ribs move inward, and the belly draw back—a full, releasing out-breath.

5. Carry on: Inhale slower and fuller, exhale longer and lighter—always comfortable, never forced.

6. Keep your attention lightly on the movement of breath and the felt sense in the body; when the mind wanders, return kindly to the breath.

7. Continue for six to ten minutes, then let the breath return to its natural rhythm and sit for a minute, noticing the change in mind and body.

**Note:* Exhalations relax, so make them longer than the inhalations but only by a comfortable length; do not force them. No breath retention is needed in this exercise. The emphasis is on the depth and slowness of the breath, not on holding it. Quality over quantity: better a few calm and full breaths than many forced ones.

Caution: If you feel lightheaded, reduce the depth or return to normal breathing. Those with respiratory or cardiovascular concerns should practice gently and consult a teacher or physician.

Closing reflection: As you finish, sit quietly and notice what has changed within you. Does your breath feel softer, your thoughts a little slower, your mood a bit lighter? This gentle calm isn't something you created—it was always there, waiting beneath the noise, revealed each time breath and awareness moved together.

4

Prāṇa Vāyus

JUST AS THE FRAGRANCE RESIDES WITHIN THE FLOWER,
SO TOO THE SELF RESIDES WITHIN THE PRĀṆA.
—YOGAVĀSIṢṬHA 6.25.61

TO BETTER UNDERSTAND prāṇa's multidimensional role in depth, the Yoga and Āyurveda traditions offer a refined framework—one that reveals how this singular life force expresses itself in diverse ways.

THE FIVE PRIMARY VĀYUS: VITAL FORCES THAT ANIMATE LIFE

There are five primary expressions of prāṇa, known as the *pancha prāṇas* or, more specifically, *pancha vāyus*, where *pancha* means "five" and *vāyu* means "wind," indicating movement. These vāyus are not separate entities, but five distinct modes of the same prāṇa, as the *Praśna Upaniṣad*

(2.3) clearly states. A helpful analogy would be that of electricity powering different appliances, like the fan, light, or pump, each performing a different task but all drawing from the same current. In addition, there are five secondary, or assistant, vāyus.

The yogic sages mapped these vāyus not as metaphorical abstractions but as directly perceivable flows of energy that can be refined, balanced, and consciously guided through yogic practices. The five primary vāyus are *prāṇa*, *apāna*, *samāna*, *udāna*, and *vyāna*, and the five secondary vāyus are *nāga, kūrma, kṛkala, devadatta,* and *dhanañjaya* (*Vedāntasāra* 84).

Each of these vāyus plays a unique role, much like the departments within an organization. Together, they form the subtle physiological infrastructure that supports metabolic processes, from respiration and digestion to communication, cognition, and elimination.

In this chapter, we briefly explore the primary and secondary prāṇa vāyus—their directions, functions, origins, and roles within the frameworks of Yoga and Āyurveda. The aim is to deepen our understanding of prāṇa as a bridge between spiritual growth and psychophysiological well-being.

Prāṇa Vāyu: Inhalation—The Wisdom of Receiving

Prāṇa vāyu governs respiration, ingestion of food, heartbeat, and sensory input. Like the intake department in an organization that handles incoming messages, energy, and materials crucial for its functioning, this vāyu facilitates what comes into the system—be it air, food, thoughts, or emotions. Its seat is the head, heart, and chest area.

According to the *Suśruta Saṃhitā—Nidānasthāna* (1.12), it holds a central and controlling role by energizing the body and the other vāyus, remaining active at all times. It is so vital that if its flow is blocked or stopped, life itself may come to an end. When it flows freely and vibrantly, it awakens harmony in the body-mind complex and noble qualities like courage, compassion, and inner knowledge. It is said to carry the energy of the Ātman—the True Self—which is said to reside in the heart.

Before we rise from a seated or lying position, we instinctively take an in-breath. This subtle act reflects the *awakening* power of prāṇa vāyu. As the *Chāndogya Upaniṣad* (1.3.6) beautifully affirms, "It is by prāṇa that all things rise." Whether it is the body lifting itself or consciousness rising to higher states, prāṇa vāyu is the vital impulse behind every upward movement, every awakening.

Every time we breathe in, we are not merely drawing in oxygen, we are giving permission to receive life, welcome possibility, and invite the energy needed to move forward and grow. In that sense, inhaling is the very act of saying yes to life. It can also be understood beyond the context of respiration—as the way we take in the world through our senses. Sights, sounds, smells, thoughts, and impressions all *enter* through this inner movement of prāṇa vāyu. The mind builds its reality from what is received in this way, and the quality of our life is ultimately shaped by what we choose to allow into our inner space.

Just before every in-breath there is a quiet, natural pause, a subtle moment in which the deeper self chooses to let life in. In that single, unspoken gesture, we open ourselves to possibility, to renewal, and to the unfolding of what comes next. Inhalation, as a function of prāṇa vāyu, is our acceptance to all that life has to offer.

When prāṇa vāyu is balanced, the breath flows smoothly and effortlessly, reflecting an inner harmony between body and mind. There is also a felt sense of lightness in the chest, courage in the heart, and resilience in daily activity, symptoms of a harmonious physiology and psychology. In a broad sense, prāṇa vāyu's functionality can be correlated with many biological functions, mainly the autonomic nervous system's control of the cardiorespiratory system and the sensory afferent pathways that bring information from the environment to the brain.

Apāna Vāyu: Exhalation—The Wisdom of Release

The term *apa* in *apāna* means "away from" or "downward," reflecting its role as the outward-moving and descending force. It governs the elimination of respiratory and metabolic byproducts through exhalation and downward or expulsive processes such as defecation, urination, menstruation, ejaculation, and childbirth. Like the sanitation or waste-management department in a city, it clears out what the system no longer needs, maintaining internal purity.

At the physical level, apāna vāyu functions in the pelvic region, between the navel and the perineum, supporting the vital activities of the kidneys, bladder, bowels, and the excretory and reproductive organs. At a subtle level, apāna plays a crucial role in the awakening of kuṇḍalinī, which lies dormant within its domain. Mastery over apāna is also said to be linked to mastery over sexual instinct, making it essential for cultivating *brahmacarya*—a disciplined channeling of vital energy toward spiritual growth.

Every time we exhale, sigh, urinate, defecate, or even vomit, we are engaging apāna vāyu. Through these actions, the body releases what it no longer needs. In this way, both exhalation and elimination become natural expressions of apāna's deeper purpose: letting go, release.

Imagine carrying heavy grocery bags across the parking lot. Your body is tense and fully engaged in effort, while your breath becomes short and rapid as you carry the load. The moment you finally set the bags down in the trunk of your car, there's a natural *aaahh*—a long, satisfying exhale. That release is apāna vāyu in action. Every act of letting go is instinctively linked to exhalation—whether it's a deeply satisfying trip to the bathroom, that irritating sneeze that finally comes out, a relieved sigh when a stressful task is over, or even a loud scream of frustration. The body *knows* how to release, and it does so through exhalation. Just as metabolic waste must be expelled to keep the body healthy, the breath too releases tension, heat, and emotional pressure. Physiologically, exhalation activates the parasympathetic nervous system, slowing the heart rate and signaling the body to relax, restoring a sense of safety and ease. That's why we often feel lighter, calmer, and more at ease after acts that are aided by exhalation. One could say that apāna vāyu represents the wisdom of release, the body's natural rhythm of cleansing, and the mind's quiet invitation to surrender.

Apāna vāyu's function could be correlated with respiratory exhalation, the enteric nervous system, parasympathetic outflow, and pelvic organ functions including the excretory and reproductive systems.

Samāna Vāyu: Harmonization— The Wisdom of Processing

Sama means "equalizing" and therefore, samāna vāyu means the equalizing or assimilatory force. It coordinates the upward movement of prāṇa vāyu and the downward movement of apāna vāyu, and in this sense it generates a sort of a vortex around the navel that results in a churning movement. Its seat is the navel, and its main function is to process, assimilate, and distribute energy, both physical and mental. It governs not only the digestion of food but also the assimilation of sensory impressions, emotions, and thoughts. Acting as a harmonizing force, it maintains balance and equilibrium in body and mind—gathering energy rather than letting it scatter. It is like the processing department in a factory that takes in raw materials and transforms them into usable products. It governs digestion, metabolism, and even mental assimilation.

The Āyurveda text *Suśruta Saṃhitā—Nidānasthāna* (1.16) says that the samāna vāyu moves in (and governs) the stomach and the region of the intestines. Its function is to digest the chyme brought down into the intestines by uniting it with the digestive fire (*jāṭharāgni*) and separating its essence from the waste products.

In yogic practice, a balanced samāna vāyu is considered essential for a strong *agni*—inner fire—which is considered necessary for efficient metabolism and energy extraction from everything that is consumed, may it be food or thought. It also fuels the inner zest, motivation, and resilience that sustain one's spiritual practice and keep the focus steady through life's challenges.

It is analogous to the integrated functioning of the enteric nervous system and intestinal absorption mechanisms that facilitate digestion and nutrient assimilation. Psychologically, it parallels the executive cognitive functions involved in processing, integration, and emotional regulation essential for mental clarity and adaptive response.

Udāna Vāyu: The Wisdom of Ascension

In Sanskrit, *ud* means "upward," and therefore, udāna vāyu is the upward-moving current of energy located primarily in the region of the throat, chest, and head. It governs speech via coordinated functioning of the vocal and respiratory apparatus, thought articulation, and higher states of awareness. Physiologically, it is linked to laryngeal function, vestibular balance, and motor control of voluntary movement.

The *Suśruta Saṃhitā—Nidānasthāna* (1.14) states that when udāna vāyu works ineffectively, it brings on diseases that are confined to regions above the clavicles. The *Praśna Upaniṣad* (3.9) mentions that it governs higher states of consciousness and upward movement of the subtle body at the time of death, guiding it to different realms as per yogic cosmology.

One could equate it to the public relations or communication team in an organization, since it enables expression and outward sharing of what's internal.

It correlates with the vocal cords and also parts of the prefrontal cortex related to self-expression and long-term memory.

Vyāna Vāyu: Circulation—The Wisdom of Diffusion

From a yogic standpoint, vyāna vāyu is considered an all-pervading force that governs the distribution of energy from the core to the periphery of the body. It is located throughout the entire body and supports circulation of blood, lymph, and neural impulses. It also aids in perspiration and five types of bodily movements: expanding, contracting, lowering down, lifting up, and lateral rising. Its disharmony leads to disease in multiple organs (*Suśruta Saṃhitā—Nidānasthāna* 1.15). This vāyu functions like the logistics and distribution team in an organization; it connects and coordinates the entire system. It correlates with the circulatory system, peripheral nervous system, and the sense of musculoskeletal coordination.

THE SECONDARY PRĀṆA VĀYUS

According to the text called *Vedāntasāra* (85), there are five secondary prāṇa vāyus—namely, nāga, which causes vomiting or erection; kūrma, which opens the eyelids; kṛkala, which creates hunger; devadatta, which produces yawning; and dhanañjaya, which is responsible for nourishing or maintaining the body. The *Yoga Chūḍāmaṇi Upaniṣad* (26) states that dhanañjaya prāṇa does not leave the body immediately after death, unlike the other vāyus, which depart at the time of death.

Each of the vāyus expresses itself in the body through different physical, mental, and energetic roles. When they work together in balance, they express themselves as good digestion, clear thinking, emotional steadiness, and a natural sense of direction in life. This harmony reflects the yogic understanding that life isn't made of separate parts but is one continuous, living flow.

BREATH AS A WAY HOME TO OURSELVES

As we study the many movements and functions of the vāyus, it's easy to start thinking of them as something mechanical happening inside us. But the truth is much simpler and deeper: we breathe not just to stay alive but to return to ourselves.

Behind every breath, there is the one who breathes. Circulation of prāṇa is not just a bodily process; it is the living pulse of who we are.

In the *Bṛhadāraṇyaka Upaniṣad* (3.4.1), the sage Yājñavalkya reminds his student Uṣasta that the embodied self is the one that breathes through prāṇa. It's the self that moves downward as apāna, spreads as vyāna, and rises as udāna. In other words, the individual self is expressed through every breath we take.

When we see this clearly, breathing becomes more than an automatic act. Each breath, each physiological function, becomes a gentle reminder—a way of coming home to our own presence in body and mind. Prāṇa is no longer just some energy moving within us; it is the intimate rhythm calling us back, again and again, to ourselves.

It is astonishing to see how modern science is now confirming what the ancient yogis intuitively understood: Each person's breath is intimately linked with their individual self. Researchers at the Weizmann Institute of Science recently discovered that every individual has a unique nasal airflow pattern, almost like a fingerprint.[10] Using a device that measures nasal airflow, they were able to identify individuals with 96.8 percent accuracy based solely on their breathing pattern—a remarkable validation of the yogic insight that the breath is deeply personal and expressive of one's inner being.

THE PRĀṆA BODY

In modern Yoga, the body is often viewed through the lens of empirical science as a system defined by anatomy, biology, and measurable functions. While this view has its value, traditional Yoga reminds us that human beings are far more than physical matter. It sees the body as a living field of energy, shaped and sustained by breath, mind, and awareness—known as the *sūkṣma śarīra*, or subtle body, also called the prāṇic body. Because of this, over the course of Yoga history, different traditions have offered varied models of the subtle body, each shaped by its own aims, practices, and philosophies. These models are not rigid anatomical structures but living frameworks cultivated through direct experience and inner exploration.

The subtle body framework is primarily comprised of a vast network of nāḍīs, prāṇa channels. As for their exact number, texts do not always present a consistent view, but the *Bṛhadāraṇyaka Upaniṣad* (2.1.19) and others state that there are seventy-two thousand nāḍīs. Yet, out of these, three are considered primary: *iḍā*, *piṅgalā*, and *suṣumnā*. The iḍā nāḍī, associated with lunar, cooling energy, flows along the left of the spine, and the piṅgalā nāḍī, with solar, activating energy, flows on the right. The suṣumnā nāḍī, the central channel aligned with the spinal column, is the most vital, as it is through this pathway that the latent kuṇḍalinī energy must rise for full spiritual awakening to occur.

Kuṇḍalinī is the individualized form of the universal creative energy (*śakti*), a latent, divine force coiled at the base of the spine in every human being. It is the potential of the Universal Consciousness itself, waiting to be awakened in the individual. In Indic traditions, kuṇḍalinī is not seen merely as an energetic force but as a goddess and a mother (*mātā*). When roused through yogic practices, "she" rises through the central channel (suṣumnā), ascending through each cakra, gradually dissolving the veils of limited identity. This ascent is not just energetic; it's a journey of expansion of consciousness via profound body–mind transformation, ultimately leading to the realization of one's unity with Universal Consciousness (Śiva), the source of all existence.

The cakras, often described as energy centers or wheels, are subtle focus points for meditation along the central channel and correspond to specific psychoenergetic states. These cakras, typically six, as stated in the *Netratantra* (5.3.1), correspond to five elements and the mind and thus govern physiological and mental functions and elemental patterns.

Yoga practices purify nāḍīs, regulate prāṇa, and guide the passage of kuṇḍalinī through the suṣumnā, piercing each cakra along the way until it merges with *sahasrāra*, the thousand-petaled lotus at the crown of the head. In this way, the subtle body becomes the vehicle of transformation, allowing the practitioner to transcend limited identity and experience the fullness of being.

A helpful modern scientific analogy for kuṇḍalinī, cakras, and nāḍīs is the electrical system of a building. Think of kuṇḍalinī as the main power source, a vast reserve of energy stored in the basement, not yet tapped to its full potential. The nāḍīs are like electrical wiring, running through the walls, carrying power to various parts of the building. The cakras are the circuit breakers or power panels on different floors, each regulating and distributing energy for specific functions: lighting, heating, communication, etc. When the wiring (nāḍīs) is clear and uncorroded and the panels (cakras) are properly tuned, the stored energy (kuṇḍalinī) can be safely and gradually released upward through the central conduit (suṣumnā), lighting up each floor (cakra) until it reaches the top level, symbolizing higher awareness or self-realization. Just as a surge in electrical current must be well-regulated to avoid short-circuiting the system, kuṇḍalinī's awakening requires purification, preparation, reverence, faith, and guidance for it to uplift rather than overwhelm.

With the sustained practice of mental concentration in prāṇāyāma, it becomes possible to *sense* and even *inwardly see* the movement of prāṇa flowing through the nāḍīs. In the early stages of practice, with closed eyes, this visual may appear as a flickering, unsteady glow, much like a flash of lightning illuminating the night sky: radiant, but brief. As the ability to concentrate deepens, the vision becomes more stable and refined. Numerous nāḍīs can be *seen* the moment one closes one's eyes, each shimmering as phosphorescent channels of varying hues depending on the nature, momentum, and clarity of the prāṇa they carry. Their structure is precise, yet they are not sensed as solid tubes—more like subtle strands of light rather than physical cords.

Blockages in the nāḍīs can result in emotional disturbances, physical ailments, or spiritual stagnation. The practitioner can become aware of prāṇic blockages within the nāḍī network too. They are perceived as areas of discoloration or opacity—darker, denser patches indicating deeper energetic obstructions. The practitioner initially regulates the flow of prāṇa through *bandhas* (intentional muscular locks) and mudrās (energetic gestures or seals), using the physical body as a means to channel the life force. With continued practice and refinement, however, this control becomes internal—guided directly by focused intention, without the need for physical manipulation.

In traditional Haṭha Yoga, these skills are cultivated for the purpose of purifying the nāḍīs, modulating the flow of prāṇa, and aiding kuṇḍalinī to ascend. As one's capacity to direct and refine the movement of inner prāṇa increases, it naturally influences the state of mind, for the two are inseparable. As kuṇḍalinī rises, the deeper layers of mind are stirred. This stirring brings to the surface old memories, primal conditioning, limiting impressions, and unresolved tendencies, all of which may not be pleasant and yet must be encountered, resolved, and integrated by the practitioner—as stated in the *Jñānēśvarī* (6.216).[11] This is what makes authentic yogic inner work both transformative and demanding, and this is also why such practices should be undertaken only with able guidance.

Since the subtle body is woven from prāṇa itself, it naturally carries the inherent qualities of prāṇa, i.e., consciousness, intelligence, movement, and connectivity. It is not a passive structure but a living, responsive field that reflects the dynamic nature of life force. This is why the prāṇic body is both the carrier and the expression of inner awakening.

Note: Just like working with electricity, working with kuṇḍalinī is subtle and powerful and requires care. The mechanics of kuṇḍalinī rising has its own inner language, procedure, and logic, much like how electricians understand the principles and precautions when it comes to wiring and handling electrical current. For this reason, kuṇḍalinī-related practices must be approached with deep faith, steadiness, and detachment and under the guidance of an authentic guru who is rooted in a living lineage and has traversed the path through direct, embodied experience rather than mere theoretical understanding.

PRĀṆA–APĀNA: THE CYCLE OF LIFE

The ancient yogis, especially the Haṭha Yoga masters, placed great emphasis on the union of prāṇa and apāna, considering it the true accomplishment (*siddhi*) of Yoga. As texts such as the *Gorakṣaśataka* (52) and *Yoga Bīja* (110) indicate, practices like prāṇāyāma and bandha are designed specifically to bring these two opposing currents together. For the Haṭha yogis, the balance of prāṇa vāyu and apāna vāyu was far more than respiratory regulation; it reflected a deeper stilling of the push and pull of life.

As we know, prāṇa vāyu is the energy of receiving and rising, while apāna vāyu is the energy of releasing and emptying. We constantly move between these two forces in our everyday life—taking in and letting go, wanting and rejecting, engaging and withdrawing. When we remain confined within this relentless exchange, we become trapped in the cycle of saṃsāra, slowly depleting our inner vitality and reinforcing separation and suffering.

The yogic insight, therefore, was not simply to balance prāṇa vāyu and apāna vāyu as respiratory breaths, but to *unite* them. In Haṭha Yoga, *Ha* refers to prāṇa and *ṭha* to apāna. *Haṭha* literally means the joining of two opposing forces. Their union enables the ascent of kuṇḍalinī, lifting the practitioner beyond duality and resting them in the unitary experience of the True Self. In this sense, the gross breath becomes a subtle gateway: Every inhale and exhale becomes an invitation to move beyond the cycle of action and reaction, rising and falling, into the steadiness of being.

Once, my teacher—who was a Siddha, a self-realized master of Yoga—quietly grinned when I asked him about prāṇa and apāna and simply said in Hindi, "*Ānā–jānā*"—literally "coming and going." It was his wordplay and a gentle way of shifting my attention beyond the technicality of breathing, reminding me that as long as these two forces remain separate, we stay caught in the endless traffic of transmigration. With his remark he pointed me to the deeper aim of Yoga: to be balanced in the dualities of life and realize the True Self.

ENDING INSIGHT

In exploring the prāṇa vāyus and the sūkṣma śarīra, we begin to glimpse the profound intelligence embedded within our very being. These ancient models remind us that we are not just a body or a mind but living energy—constantly moving, feeling, and responding in rhythm with life. The yogic seers saw the body not as a material machine but as a vibrant field of consciousness, alive with purpose and potential. At every moment, billions of physiological processes unfold within us in perfect coordination—the heart beating, lungs expanding, neurons firing, enzymes activating—each system communicating and depending on the other in silent intelligence. The nervous, circulatory, digestive, and lymphatic systems all move in a delicate dance of interdependence, guided by an organizing awareness that science can describe but not fully explain. The vāyus are expressions of this very organizing awareness within us—subtle movements that shape how we breathe, act, think, and grow. When we learn to understand and balance these energies, they become steady companions in our journey of inner awakening.

The subtle body, composed of prāṇa, is not separate from who we are; it is the bridge between the seen and unseen, the outer world and the Inner Self. In honoring and working with subtle anatomy, we honor life as sacred movement—within and beyond breath.

Prāṇāyāma Practice: The Meeting of Prāṇa and Apāna

To experience the living rhythm of life through the simple awareness of inhalation and exhalation, the meeting of prāṇa vāyu (the current of receiving) and apāna vāyu (the current of releasing), do the following:

Instructions

1. **Position:** Sit with the spine straight and eyes gently closed. Let the body relax and settle into stillness, and let the breath return to its own quiet rhythm.

2. **Awareness of inhalation:** As you breathe in, sense the gentle rising movement of prāṇa vāyu—the energy flowing in through your nose and upward toward the heart and chest—drawing in vitality, clarity, and light. Keep the inhale easy, do not deepen it. Simply *witness* how life enters you.

3. **Awareness of exhalation:** As you breathe out, feel the downward and outward settling of apāna vāyu—the natural movement of release, grounding, and letting go. Let the body soften and the mind relax.

4. **Meeting point:** Notice the brief, silent, natural pause between inhale and exhale—a moment where prāṇa and apāna meet and merge. This is not a pause you create or control nor a holding of the breath but a natural still point that arises on its own. Rest your awareness there, where movement becomes stillness. In that stillness between two

breaths lies the doorway to timelessness—a silence that is not empty but full of presence. Tune in to the sacred quiet of this pause, where the mind becomes naturally still.

5. **Continuation**: Remain with this simple awareness of inhale, exhale, and pause for several rounds of breath. Let each inhalation lift, each exhalation settle, and each pause make you still—like the tides of the ocean, effortlessly sustaining life. Let each pause be a return to the source, a reminder of the still center within which all motion turns.

6. **Completion**: Allow the breath to continue on its own for ten minutes or as long as the breath remains effortless. Sit quietly for a few moments, sensing how every breath is the union of ascent and descent, receiving and releasing—the pulse of existence itself.

5

Prāṇic Practices

The uniting of the prāṇa, the mind, and the senses—
detachment from conditional existence.
This is called Yoga.
—Maitri Upaniṣad 6.25

Now that we understand prāṇa more deeply, it's clear that working with prāṇa goes far beyond simple breathwork. The ancient yogic seers devised a vast and nuanced array of prāṇa-based practices to deepen awareness of its presence and to master its movement for physical, mental, and spiritual well-being. These practices were meant for all—laypeople, householders, and ascetics alike. In light of this larger vision, we now turn to the diverse prāṇa-based practices found across Indic spiritual traditions. To bring clarity to the spectrum of prāṇic practices, I present a twofold classification. This is not a traditional bifurcation but a simplified framework offered here to help modern seekers navigate the various ways in which Indic thought has approached prāṇa.

1. **Prāṇa upāsanā:** *Upāsanā* means "sitting near with reverence" and refers to devotional and contemplative approaches to prāṇa through outward engagements, rituals, visualizations, prayers, a disciplined lifestyle, and a conscious connection with natural forces like the Sun, wind, fire, and Moon. These practices cultivate sensitivity, deepen reverence, and attune the practitioner to prāṇa's presence in the world.

2. **Prāṇa āyāma:** *Āyāma* means "expansion" or "extension," and when joined with the prefix prāṇa, it forms the term *prāṇāyāma*. It refers to the inward modulation and refinement of prāṇa through breath control, cleansing practices, mantra repetition, physical movement, and focused awareness. It includes techniques that help regulate the flow of prāṇa within the body–mind complex, supporting inner balance, vitality, and spiritual transformation.

Together, these approaches offer a holistic path to cultivating inner and outer harmony through conscious engagement with prāṇa. Let us now explore these time-honored approaches and their significance.

PRĀṆA UPĀSANĀ: THE OUTWARD PRĀṆA PRACTICES

Over time, many practices arose as prāṇa upāsanā that honor the sacred presence of prāṇa through worship, visualization, elemental reverence, and consecration. Let's explore a few of them.

Prāṇa Pratiṣṭhā: Prāṇa, the Bridge from Stone to Sacred

Prāṇa pratiṣṭhā means "establishment of life force." It is the sacred ritual of infusing life (prāṇa) into an idol (*murti*), thereby transforming it from a mere sculpture into a living embodiment of the deity worthy of worship (*Kālikā Purāṇa* 88.15–16). Through this ritual, performed in temples and homes, the statue or image is enlivened into a vibrant deity capable of receiving prayers and bestowing blessings.

This ritual reflects the deeper metaphysical understanding that prāṇa is the very link between consciousness and matter. Just as prāṇa enlivens our physical body and enables self-awareness, the prāṇa pratiṣṭhā ritual enlivens the idol and makes the presence of the deity accessible to the devotee's heart. Once consecrated with prāṇa, the idol is no longer just an object of stone or metal; it becomes a living expression of the divine presence. From that moment, the deity is felt to be truly alive—watching, guiding, and blessing the devotee. For the devotee, the idol is not a symbol but the living form of the divine they love and worship.

This is why, in the Hindu tradition, visiting a temple is not considered merely a "temple visit"; it is called *darśana*—the act of sacred seeing. One is not simply looking at a temple deity's idol but encountering a living presence, awakened through prāṇic exchange between the deity and the devotee. It is a moment of mutual connection—the devotee sees and is seen, touched inwardly by the living prāṇa within the idol. Prāṇa bridges the distance between them, turning devotion into a living relationship.

Such acts of faith and prāṇic communion can be deeply healing. They soothe the heart, steady the mind, and lift us beyond fear, loneliness, and the ache of feeling unseen. In the quiet space between the devotee and the consecrated idol, prāṇa becomes the invisible bridge—the living current that carries love, devotion, trust, and presence in both directions. This is how prāṇa becomes an integral aspect of Bhakti Yoga. Through this shared breath of life, Bhakti Yoga reveals its depth: It is not merely worship of an external form but a communion of energies where the prāṇa of the devotee aligns with the prāṇa awakened in the deity. In this connection, faith is no longer belief alone; it becomes a felt experience of being held, guided, and renewed by the same living force that moves through all existence.

Prāṇa Upāsanā of Deities like Sun, Moon, and Fire

In the ancient Indian worldview, celestial forces such as the Sun (Sūrya) and Moon (Candra) were not seen merely as physical phenomena but as living embodiments of prāṇa. These celestial bodies were seen as sources of light, nourishment, rhythm, and healing—deeply linked to both personal and collective well-being. For this reason, ancient yogis developed practices of reverence and contemplation to connect with and draw in the cosmic prāṇa that flows through all of creation.

Sūrya upāsanā, the worship of the Sun, is a central prāṇic practice, with hymns dedicated to the Sun found throughout the *Ṛg Veda* (notably the *Sūrya Sūkta*, *Ṛg Veda* 1.50) and also the powerful *Āditya Hṛdayam* from the *Valmīki Rāmāyaṇa* (6.105), where the Sun is invoked as the remover of sorrow and bestower of strength, clarity, and vitality. Sūrya upāsanā is performed at different times of the day by offering libation (*arghya*) and chanting mantras for the practitioner's well-being and prosperity. On Amāvasyā (the new Moon), Candra upāsanā—worship of the Moon—is performed to invoke blessings for progeny and relief from sorrow.

Such forms of worship show how simple acts of reverence and gratitude can connect us to something vast and living. When we engage with the flow of cosmic prāṇa in this way, we awaken a quiet strength within and begin to feel in harmony with the larger rhythm of life itself.

Fire worship and fire rituals (*yajñas*) are among the most sacred acts in the Vedic tradition. Fire (agni) is seen not merely as one of the five elements but as a living presence infused with prāṇa. The same fire that burns as the Sun also burns within us, sustaining life and linking all beings in one cosmic flow of energy. In Vedic rituals, the fire altar (*yajña kuṇḍa*) represents the human body itself, with the five prāṇas invoked as its vital forces. Through this symbolism, agni becomes the sacred bridge between the cosmic and the personal—aligning human life with the rhythm of the divine (*Praśna Upaniṣad* 4.3). Revered as the *sākṣī*, the silent witness, agni mirrors the same awareness that watches within us—the inner fire of consciousness that sees without judgment and transforms through its very presence.

Eating as Prāṇa Upāsanā

There is a beautiful concept in the Vedic tradition called *prāṇa agnihotra* (*Chāndogya Upaniṣad* 5.19.1), which talks about turning the outer fire ritual inward. In this understanding, the simple act of eating becomes a sacred offering—the food we take in is like an oblation poured into the inner fire of digestion (*jāṭharāgni*). Through this awareness, nourishment becomes worship, and every meal turns into an act of gratitude.

Many years ago, during my study in an āśrama, we practiced a simple yet deeply meaningful ritual before every meal called *ācamanam*—the act of sipping or sprinkling water to symbolically purify the mouth, senses, and body. Accompanied by quiet mantras and mindful gestures, this ritual is said to prepare the body and mind to receive food as sacred prāṇic nourishment. The *Chāndogya Upaniṣad* (5.2.2) beautifully calls water the "clothing of prāṇa," suggesting that it sanctifies prāṇa in the food for the process of digestion. In this seemingly ordinary act, eating becomes a sacred ritual—where each bite is received with gratitude and the act of eating itself becomes a prayer. As the meal ends, a final sip of water is taken, "clothes prāṇa," completing the sacred cycle in reverence.

In this way, when we begin to see through the wider vision of prāṇa, even something as ordinary as eating becomes sacred—for we sense the same life force moving through the food, the breath, and ourselves. Can we pause for just a breath before eating and marvel at this living exchange of prāṇa? What if every meal became an opportunity to feel grateful for the ways life keeps us alive?

Diet and Lifestyle Moderation as Prāṇa Upāsanā

In yogic thought, developing harmony in diet and lifestyle is seen as a prāṇic practice. Just as mindful breathing harmonizes prāṇa, mindful intake of food, aligned with daily rhythms, also harmonizes prāṇa. This is why diet (*āhāra*) and daily routine (*dinacaryā*) are considered foundational pillars of Āyurveda and Yoga.

Ancient yogis knew about the delicate relationship between food and mind. The *Chāndogya Upaniṣad* (7.26.2) says, "If one eats pure food, one's mind becomes pure. If the mind is pure, one's memory becomes strong and steady. If the memory is good, one becomes free from all bondage."

The prāṇa we receive from food is influenced not just by what we eat but also by how, when, and in what state of mind we eat. Fresh, minimally processed, *sāttvika* foods are believed to carry more prāṇa. The mindset during cooking and eating—whether calm, grateful, or distracted—also affects how prāṇa is transmitted and absorbed in the cooked food. Eating in alignment with one's constitution, digestive capability, and daily rhythms enhances assimilation, making the act of eating not just a physical act but a powerful prāṇa-cultivation practice. This is why the *Gheraṇḍa Saṃhitā* (5.2) emphasizes that the essential prerequisites for beginning the practice of prāṇāyāma are moderation of diet (*mitāhāra*) and cleansing of the nāḍīs (*nāḍī śuddhi*). Without these foundational preparations, the subtle regulation of prāṇa is neither stable nor effective.

Dinacaryā is the lifestyle component. Our habits directly influence the flow and quality of prāṇa by affecting our nervous system, breath patterns, and biological rhythms.

Irregular sleep, excessive screen time, or sedentary behavior can disrupt prāṇic balance, leading to fatigue or mental agitation. Daily routines such as timely exercise, eating, sleeping, managing screen time, sufficient rest, the right amount of effort, and aligning with the natural cycles of the seasons (*ṛtus*) and time (*kāla*) help preserve prāṇic rhythm. Studies show that consistent lifestyle habits improve vagal tone and heart rate variability[12]—both indicators of balanced autonomic function and subtle energy regulation. This is why yogic texts like the *Bhagavad Gītā* (6.17) and the *Haṭha Yoga Pradīpikā* (1.57) emphasize moderation in eating, sleeping, and lifestyle as essential for success in Yoga.

When we bring awareness to daily choices, even the simplest habits like eating and resting take on a deeper significance. What if we began to see diet and lifestyle not merely as mechanical means for attaining physical well-being but as prāṇa upāsanā—conscious prāṇic rituals with the power to shape the state of our mind and the quality of our life?

Prāṇa Pratyāropaṇa as Prāṇa Upāsanā: Transmission of Sacred Prāṇa

Prāṇa pratyāropaṇa refers to the conscious transference of prāṇaśakti—prāṇic energy—from one being to another, most often from a teacher (guru) or parent to a worthy disciple or child. Rooted in the Indian spiritual tradition, this act is performed when the guru or parent senses that their time in the physical body is drawing to a close. They are said to transmit not only their prāṇa but also their powers such as speech (*vāc*), sensory capabilities, intellect, and spiritual strength into the recipient who is capable and humble enough to receive this sacred inheritance. After the transfer, the elder renounces the world and departs, while the successor carries forward the responsibility of ensuring the unbroken flow of higher spiritual purpose and vision (*paramārtha*).

This profound act can also happen in sacred transmissions like initiation (*dīkṣā*) and the infusion of spiritual energy (*śaktipāta*). In these acts, the guru doesn't merely give instruction; they become the channel for awakened prāṇa, transferring it directly into the disciple through touch, thought, mantra, gaze, dreams, or even silence (*Kularnavatantra* 4.34–38). The guru's refined prāṇa carries the potency of self-realization and becomes the spark that ignites the disciple's inner transformation. More specifically, the yogis talk about something called the *ativāhika deha*, literally, "the vehicle that carries beyond the physical" (*Yogavāsiṣṭha* 6.51.50). It is the prāṇic body that enables continuity of consciousness beyond the physical form—during dreams, astral travel, or after death. Acting as a bridge between the gross body and the True Self, it allows spiritually evolved yogis to move beyond physical limitations for further spiritual evolution or to serve the world in unseen ways. Maharṣi Patañjali calls such yogis *videhas* (Yoga Sūtra 1.19).

Prāṇa pratyāropaṇa represents the highest expression of prāṇa upāsanā, where one's own prāṇic energy is offered as an instrument to uplift others, to sustain the flame of spiritual knowledge, and to keep the current of dharma alive across generations. This sacred act reaffirms the Indian understanding of prāṇa not just as a biological force but as the vehicle of dharma, wisdom, and spiritual continuity.

Prāṇa Upāsanā Through Swara Vidyā: The Science of Breath Manipulation

The ancient yogis developed a highly refined system of breath awareness and control known as *swara vidyā*. Here, *swara* denotes the subtle flow of prāṇa vāyu through the nostrils and nāḍīs. Rooted in texts like the *Śiva Swarodaya* and *Pavana Vijaya Swarodaya*, this knowledge system outlines how the alternating flow of breath through the iḍā and piṅgalā channels influence one's physical energy, mental clarity, emotional state, and the outcome of daily activities. Yogis, warriors, priests, traders, and healers traditionally used the wisdom of swara to choose the right time for action, rest, battle, negotiations, and trade; to enhance success; and to manage their life. By consciously observing and, at times, manipulating the breath flow, practitioners sought the alignment of cosmic rhythms, elemental influences, and mental states to gain mastery over both the subtle and gross aspects of life. Far more than mere breath observation, swara vidyā is a sacred tool for energetic discernment and modulation. As a line in the *Pavana Vijaya Swarodaya* (2.75) says, "One who masters *swara-jñāna*—the knowledge of swara—attains effortless success, even when lacking wealth."

PRĀṆĀYĀMA: THE INWARD PRĀṆA PRACTICES

Now let us look at some prāṇāyāma practices for consciously expanding, refining, and directing the flow of inner prāṇa. These include breath modalities and other powerful practices for cultivating breathing capacity, health and well-being, subtle awareness, vitality, and energetic harmony within. For ease of understanding, we will look at prāṇāyāma in four parts:

1. **Nāḍī śodhana:** Cleansing of nāḍīs
2. **Prāṇa nirodha:** Retention of breath
3. **Prāṇa dhāraṇā:** Concentration of prāṇa
4. **Prāṇa ūrdhvagamana:** Ascension of prāṇa

Since prāṇāyāma is conscious regulation of prāṇa, it first requires nāḍī śodhana—the cleansing of the nāḍīs—because without clear nāḍīs, prāṇa cannot be effectively moved and directed.

Nāḍī Śodhana: Cleansing the Nāḍīs

Nāḍī śodhana is the act of clearing the nāḍīs for safe, steady, and transformative prāṇic cultivation. According to the *Yoga Chūḍāmaṇi Upaniṣad* (94) and the *Gheraṇḍa Saṃhitā* (5.35), it is only when the nāḍīs are purified and prāṇa flows smoothly that the practitioner becomes capable of prāṇāyāma.

Without cleansed nāḍīs, prāṇāyāma practices could lead to discomfort. Just as water flows smoothly through a pipe only when it is clear of blockages, prāṇa too can circulate effectively only when the inner pathways—the nāḍīs—are clean, steady, and balanced.

In contemporary Yoga, nāḍī śodhana is often associated with a specific breathing exercise called nāḍī śodhana prāṇāyāma, which is widely known as alternate nostril breathing and is highly praised for its balancing effect on the nervous system. However, in a broader sense of the term, nāḍī śodhana can also happen through non-breath-based practices such as *śuddhi kriyās* (organ cleansing techniques), āsana (prāṇa-guided movement and postures), mantra *japa* (devoted mantra repetition), and *dhāraṇā* (meditative awareness). Each of these practices has the potential to help dissolve energetic blockages, making the nāḍī system more refined and receptive for prāṇa to flow freely. Let us look at the different methods of nāḍī cleansing.

Śuddhi Kriyā: Organ-Cleansing-Based Nāḍī Purification

Śuddhi kriyās, or organ purification techniques, are foundational practices in the Haṭha Yoga tradition, described in classical texts such as the *Haṭha Yoga Pradīpikā* (2.22) and the *Gheraṇḍa Saṃhitā* (1.10–1.12). Techniques like *netī* (nasal cleansing), *dhautī* (cleansing of the digestive tract), *naulī* (abdominal massage through muscular churnings), *basti* (enema), *kapālabhātī* (forceful rhythmic exhalation), and *trāṭaka* (steady gazing) are designed to remove accumulated impurities (*malas*).

Physical cleansing of the mouth, nose, eyes, and other organs helps the body release what it doesn't need, bringing freshness and balance back to the system. It clears the way for prāṇa to move freely through the body and mind. Cleansing can happen through simple means—water, air, gentle friction, or specific yogic modulations. Without this inner and outer cleansing, practices like āsana or prāṇāyāma may stir up hidden impurities, sometimes causing restlessness or discomfort. Imagine trying to breathe through a blocked nose—the same thing happens when the pathways of prāṇa are not clear.

As the internal channels are cleansed, prāṇa begins to move more freely, enhancing vitality, clarity, and inner lightness. You might notice this after a simple practice like nasal cleansing—your breath feels clearer, your head lighter, and your mind more awake. Or after digestive cleansing, the heaviness lifts, leaving you feeling spacious and refreshed, as if life is flowing through you again.

Śuddhi kriyās are also said to stimulate the inner fire (agni) and prepare the body to channel and retain heightened prāṇic energy for advanced practices. Thus, śuddhi kriyās are not merely preparatory but transformational, bridging the gap between the physical body and the subtle energy field.

Āsana-, Mudrā-, and Bandha-Based Nāḍī Purification

Beyond its obvious health and postural benefits, āsana practice is also seen as a nāḍī purification technique, subtly preparing the body to become a vessel for harmoniously flowing prāṇa. Through the mindful positioning of limbs, breath, and attention, āsanas can help release muscular tension, align awareness, and balance the flow of prāṇa. Haṭha Yoga scriptures, such as the *Haṭha Yoga Pradīpikā* (1.41) and the *Haṭhatattvakaumudī* (7.51), emphatically affirm that the practice of āsana aids in the cleansing of the nāḍīs, thus playing a foundational role in preparing the body for prāṇāyāma and higher, subtler yogic practices.

Mudrās, often described as specific bodily gestures or energetic seals, work more subtly by creating specific prāṇic circuits in the body. When combined with focused awareness and breath, mudrās are said to purify the entire nāḍī network (*nāḍī jāla*) (*Yoga Chūḍāmaṇi Upaniṣad* [65]). Mudrās redirect and conserve prāṇa, thus promoting internal stability and mental clarity.

Bandhas (energetic locks), on the other hand, use muscular contractions to control or pool the prāṇa in specific areas, especially in the central channel (suṣumnā nāḍī), preventing its dissipation and encouraging its upward flow, as stated in the *Haṭha Yoga Pradīpikā* (3.23, 3.54). In addition to these, scriptures like the *Haṭhatattvakaumudī* and the *Siddhānta Śekhara* also prescribe specific spine, joint, and body mobilizations called *merucalana* and *cāraṇā* that cleanse the nāḍīs and are said to prepare the practitioner for prāṇāyāma. These physical practices, when done with awareness, precision, and faith, serve as gateways to inner balance, energetic harmony, and spiritual integration.

Mantra-Based Nāḍī Purification Mantra chanting is not merely a devotional act but a precise vibrational science that purifies, aligns, and empowers the prāṇic network. When practiced with firm faith (*śraddhā*) and intention (*saṅkalpa*), mantras act as a powerful tool for cleansing the nāḍīs. In both Vedic and Tantric traditions, sound (*nāda*) is regarded as the primal vibration from which the universe arises. In the *Śatapatha Brāhmaṇa* (1.4.3), the ṛṣis reveal how mantra and breath (prāṇa) are intrinsically coordinated.

Each seed-sound (*bīja*) mantra, like *OṀ*, *HRĪṂ*, or *ŚRĪṂ*, carries a specific vibrational frequency that influences different aspects of the energetic body. Chanting these mantras repeatedly refines inner resonance, breaks through stagnation, and harmonizes the flow of prāṇa across the nāḍīs.

Some scriptures like the *Gheraṇḍa Saṃhitā* (5.37–44) talk about *Samanu Prāṇāyāma*, which combines breath regulation, mantras, visualization, and feeling or intention (*bhāvanā*) to purify the nāḍī system in a systematic way. Just like nāḍī śodhana and prāṇāyāma, mantra practices, too, should be done under the guidance of a right teacher/guru.

Nāḍī Śodhana Prāṇāyāma: Breath-Based Nāḍī Purification We now turn to how breath itself can purify the nāḍīs. As the nāḍīs clear, prāṇa flows freely, and through prāṇāyāma, even subtler blockages are released. Breath-based nāḍī cleansing modalities have been described in a variety of permutations and combinations across scriptures, including the following:

- Simple inhaling and exhaling through both nostrils
- Inhaling and exhaling through both nostrils with breath holds (*kumbhaka*)

- Inhaling and exhaling through alternate nostrils
- Inhaling through both nostrils and exhaling through one
- Inhaling and exhaling through alternate nostrils with breath holds
- Inhaling and exhaling through alternate nostrils without breath holds but with visualization and mantra contemplation
- Inhaling and exhaling through alternate nostrils with visualization but without breath holds and mantra contemplation

Kapālabhātī, often translated as "shining skull," is another dynamic, breath-based nāḍī-cleansing practice (*Haṭha Yoga Pradīpikā* 2.36, *Haṭha Tattva Kaumudī* 8.16–17). It is traditionally used to purify nāḍīs, remove metabolic waste (*āma*), and awaken dormant prāṇa. While some schools classify kapālabhātī as prāṇāyāma, others include it specifically under nāḍī śodhana due to its cleansing effects. In our classification, we place it within breath-based nāḍī purification, as it effectively serves both purposes.

A popular technique among contemporary Yoga practitioners is what is often referred to as *nāḍī śodhana prāṇāyāma* or *anuloma viloma prāṇāyāma*—the alternate nostril breath, as outlined in the *Haṭha Yoga Pradīpikā* (2.8–9). This practice involves conscious regulation of breath through alternate nostrils, optionally coupled with breath retention (kumbhaka). However, how and for how long to hold the breath depends entirely on the practitioner's physical constitution, mental steadiness, and spiritual preparedness.

The traditional masters are unanimous on one point: These practices are not to be rushed into. They are to be approached gradually, with reverence, patience, and the guidance of a qualified teacher, allowing the body–mind system to adapt and deepen naturally over time.

In the *Haṭha Yoga Pradīpikā* (2.6–2.9), author Yogi Svātmārāma clearly advises that the practice of prāṇāyāma should be undertaken with a calm and serene state of mind, in accordance with one's individual capacity, and without haste or force. Prāṇāyāma is not a performance or competition, nor a means to satisfy the ego. It is a sacred inner process that unfolds best with patience, humility, and self-awareness. Progress comes not through force but through patience, sincerity, faith, and mindful practice.

Thus, the conscious regulation of prāṇa, i.e., prāṇāyāma, rests on the foundational process of nāḍī śodhana, or purification of the nāḍīs. Through these preparatory practices, the practitioner gradually cultivates the inner clarity, breath capacity, and steadiness needed for breath retention and deeper meditative absorption.

Prāṇa Nirodha: Breath Retention

Under *prāṇa nirodha*, we will look at breath practices that work with conscious stilling or inward withdrawal of prāṇa. While in the previous sections we looked at cleansing the nāḍīs, prāṇa nirodha is where one works on stilling the restless flow of prāṇa via breath retention, or kumbhaka. These practices are essential to cultivating deeper yogic states and prepare the mind to enter single-minded concentration (*dhyāna*) and ultimately, meditative absorption (samādhi), where both the breath and thought are transcended.

Maharṣi Patañjali's definition of prāṇāyāma (Yoga Sūtra 2.49) implies breath retention, as he describes it as the practice by which the movement of the breath—inhalation (*śvāsa*) and exhalation (*praśvāsa*)—is reduced and restricted.

In prāṇāyāma practice, *recaka* refers to exhalation, and *pūraka* to inhalation. Kumbhaka is the retention of breath, which can occur either after inhalation, called inner retention (*āntara kumbhaka*), or after exhalation, called outer retention (*bahir kumbhaka*). With consistent practice, one reaches a spontaneous and effortless breath retention (*kevala kumbhaka*) that arises when the breath naturally becomes still, marking a deep internal stillness and meditative absorption. Kevala kumbhaka is the goal of breath-based yogic practices, which, in Yoga Sūtra 2.50, Maharṣi Patañjali calls *stambhavritti*, or immobilized movement. The spontaneity of kevala kumbhaka is to be reached gradually, over time, with diligent practice in slowing down the breath rate and conscious practice of breath holds.

The *Haṭha Yoga Pradīpikā* (2.44) outlines eight kumbhaka practices: *sūryabheda*, *ujjāyī*, *sītkārī*, *śītalī*, *bhastrikā*, *bhrāmarī*, *mūrcchā*, and *plāvinī*. Several other Haṭha Yoga texts like the *Gheraṇḍa Saṃhitā* (5.46) also present similar or slightly modified versions. In these practices, the breath is intentionally retained, either after inhalation or exhalation, for specific durations, with or without the use of seed mantras (bijas) and deity contemplations—often tailored to the practitioner's capacity, level, and intended outcome. In the initial stages of training, these techniques are often practiced without breath retention, allowing the body and nervous system to gradually adapt to the discipline of controlled breathing. To support and intensify the retention, bandhas such as *jālandhara*, *uḍḍiyāna*, and *mūla* are also applied if needed.

Reasons Why Yogis Practiced Breath Retention Beyond its physical benefits, breath retention (kumbhaka) held a deeper purpose for ancient yogis. They practiced breath retention not merely to strengthen the lungs but also to access subtler, deeper states of awareness. Now, let's look at some of the deeper reasons why yogis practiced it.

- **Atonement (prāyaścitta):** Retaining the breath is regarded as having powerful purifying effects, not only on the nāḍīs but also on karma. Since prāṇāyāma mainly works on the mind, and the mind is seen as the storehouse of karmic tendencies from this and past lives—it is believed that prāṇāyāma can directly influence and help balance one's karma. This is why several traditional texts recommend prāṇāyāma as a means of atonement for moral or spiritual transgressions. The *Baudhāyana Dharmasūtra* (4.1.30) states, "For destroying all faults it is this which is pre-eminent."[13] Another benefit given in scriptures like the *Haṭha Tattva Kaumudī* (12.2) is "liberation from sins (*pāpa*)" where *pāpa* refers to the accumulation of limiting karma arising from sinful, unethical, or nondharmic actions, which obstruct one's spiritual progress and well-being.
- **Tapas:** The dedicated practice of prāṇāyāma is often compared to *tapas*—the inner heat and disciplined effort needed to purify and burn away deep-seated mental impressions and obstacles. Yogis who withdrew into forests and dedicated themselves to long hours of intense prāṇāyāma and other disciplined practices, especially in the Haṭha tradition, came to be known as *tapasvīs*, those who undertake intense tapas. The term reflects not just their austerity but their unwavering commitment to inner purification and self-realization. Across thousands of years of yogic

tradition, there have been many accounts of yogis voluntarily being buried underground for days, entering a profound state of mental absorption (samādhi) while suspending the breath. Far from being a stunt, this was seen as a form of *tapasyā*—an intense spiritual discipline where the yogi withdrew completely from the external world to deepen their union with the Inner Self. In this light, breath holds (kumbhaka) are more than just physical exercises; they function as rituals of inner purification, burning away the old self to make way for the new.

- **Kuṇḍalinī awakening**: The *Haṭha Yoga Pradīpikā* (2.41) states that through consistent and systematic practice of breath retention, the nāḍīs and cakras are worked upon, allowing prāṇa to pierce open the gateway of the suṣumnā—the central channel—enabling kuṇḍalinī to enter and ascend with ease. In simple terms, when the mind is restless, prāṇa continuously oscillates between the iḍā and piṅgalā nāḍīs, preventing the arousal of kuṇḍalinī. But when the nāḍīs are cleansed, the breath becomes still, the mind grows calm, the dual currents are harmonized, and their alternating activity is transcended. This harmony allows kuṇḍalinī to awaken and rise through the suṣumnā, moving upward through the cakras, initiating deeper states of spiritual awareness and transformation.

Prāṇa-based practices form a vital part of the Yoga of Vajrayāna Buddhism too, where the practitioners focus on working with the subtle channels (*tsa-s*) and vital winds (lung-s), the Tibetan equivalent of nāḍīs and prāṇa vāyus. These practices also emphasize breath retention, visualization, and subtle awareness to activate deep transformation.

- **Mind Stilling and Subtler Practice Preparation:** Breath retention is regarded in Yoga as a powerful means of stilling the mind. As the breath is consciously inhaled, held, and released, its rhythm naturally slows, and with it, mental restlessness begins to quiet. When the breath slows, thoughts calm. When you deliberately slow down your breath, you're sending a direct "all clear" signal to your nervous system. This immediately activates your "rest and digest" mode, which is the body's natural state of calm. This easy practice dramatically reduces stress and anxiety by improving your heart rate variability—a key marker of a healthy, adaptable heart.[14] In short, slow, controlled breathing is a powerful, science-backed way to keep your heart and mind flexible, calm, and ready to handle life. Numerous scientific studies confirm that slow, deep breathing impacts brain wave activity,[15] supporting this yogic insight. A scripture by the name of *Tirumantiram* expresses this link poetically: "The mind rides on the horse of prāṇa—slow the horse, and the mind slows down" (*Tirumantiram* 564).

As the breath becomes increasingly more gentle, and the pauses between breaths grow longer, the mind naturally becomes quieter and more settled. As the internal turbulence subsides, external triggers lose their power to disturb the mind, habitual patterns (saṃskāras) begin to loosen their grip, and the mind becomes like a clear mirror, potentially ready for a direct perception of the Ātman, the True Self. This, according to Yoga Sūtras 2.52–2.53, is the real goal of prāṇāyāma.

Short breath retentions can briefly interrupt the usual flow of thoughts. As the pauses gradually deepen with practice, this stillness grows stronger—sometimes leading to a momentary quieting of the very sense of "I." In these quiet moments, all that remains is pure awareness, untouched by thought or ego. This becomes a fertile ground for experience of samādhi, which modern science would describe as an altered, nonordinary state of consciousness.

Interestingly, studies on free divers, who hold their breath for long periods of time, have shown marked psychological and neurological adaptations. In one such study, during the 6.5-minute breath hold of a free diver, the brain demonstrated a profound coping mechanism.[16] Brain imaging revealed a shift into a state resembling deep, meditative focus, marked by a surge in alpha brain waves and increased coordination within the brain's networks for introspection and visualization.

Simultaneously, the regions of the brain responsible for registering bodily sensations and discomfort became noticeably less active. This neurological pattern suggests the diver was able to temporarily mentally detach from the physical urgency and anxiety associated with breath holding, achieving an altered state of consciousness characterized by intense internal awareness and a remarkable dissociation from their physical body. These patterns closely resemble the neural signatures observed in deep meditative practices. In a yogic sense, this parallels the effects of kumbhaka, where breath retention helps suspend ordinary sensory processing and opens the doorway to altered states of consciousness, samādhi.

Breath Retention and Patience Breath retention may sound powerful and alluring, but its depth unfolds only with patience. It reveals its true value slowly, through steady and mindful practice.

The *Yogavāsiṣṭha* (5.78.46) emphasizes that breath retention brings calmness to the mind and should be cultivated through steady and patient practice (*abhyāsa*). Echoing this view, the Jain Yoga master Hemacandra, in his *Yogaśāstra* (6.2), remarks that painful or forceful methods of breath control are unnecessary, as breath mastery alone cannot lead to liberation. Similarly, the great Śaiva master Abhinavagupta, in his *Tantrāloka* (4.91), advises that prāṇāyāma should only be practiced to the extent that it does not cause discomfort (*pīḍā*).

Even Haṭha Yoga masters have emphasized the need for discernment and moderation. They insist on the right conditions like appropriate place, time, season, diet, technique, inner readiness, and, importantly, the guidance of a qualified guru, along with supportive practices like bandha, mantra, and meditation. These voices from diverse traditions together point to a shared wisdom: Prāṇāyāma must be approached with care, balance, and inner awareness.

Prāṇa Dhāraṇā: Holding Prāṇa for Meditation and Healing

Prāṇa dhāraṇā, meaning "holding prāṇa," refers to the practice of using prāṇa as the focus of meditative concentration (dhāraṇā) or focusing and redirecting prāṇa for therapeutic purposes. As for meditative concentration, the Buddhist tradition includes the *ānāpānasati* meditation, where one observes the natural flow of breath to cultivate subtle awareness, steady the mind, and awaken insight (*vipassanā*). Similar prāṇa-based meditations are also found in Tantric texts such as the *Vijñānabhairavatantra* (verse 24), where breath becomes a gateway to transcendental awareness.

Beyond meditative concentration, yogic scriptures like the *Darśanopaniṣad* (6.24) and the *Triśikhibrāhmaṇa Upaniṣad* (110) describe methods of directing and holding prāṇa in specific regions, such as the heart, tip of the nose, navel, or forehead, by concentrating awareness there and increasing or decreasing the prāṇa flow in that region. This purposeful redirection of prāṇa serves therapeutic functions, aiding in healing, removing energetic blockages (granthis), and enhancing vitality in affected areas. The *Haṭha Tattva Kaumudī* (12.12) even notes that prāṇa dhāraṇā can help overcome premature death. The *Bṛhadāraṇyaka Upaniṣad* (1.3.28) praises meditation on prāṇa as one of the highest practices, saying that through it, one can "win the world." When we meditate on prāṇa, it stops feeling separate from us; we begin to sense it as our very essence—the force that moves, sustains, and finally leads us back to the stillness of the True Self that it comes from.

Thus, prāṇa dhāraṇā emerges as a profound meditative and therapeutic discipline, rooted in awareness, empowered by intention, and aimed at inner transformation.

So'Ham: When Breath Itself Becomes the Mantra

Through their holistic vision, the ancient yogis discovered a practice so simple yet so profoundly transformative that it turns every breath into a mantra and every moment into a prayer. It is a multidimensional practice—seen through the lens of breath, it is prāṇāyāma; through the lens of awareness, it becomes meditation; and through the lens of devotion, it turns into japa, the sacred repetition of divine remembrance. Yogis call this practice *ajapā*, the "non-japa," because the mantra is neither spoken by the tongue nor deliberately repeated in the mind. It is an effortless awareness that arises on its own, flowing naturally with the rhythm of the breath. Here's how the process of ajapā unfolds.

The seers observed that hidden within each breath lies a subtle mantra. Our inhalation produces a soft *sa* sound, and our exhalation a gentle *ha*—the sound of a sigh, of release, of surrender. When Sanskrit phonetic rules are applied, *sa* and *ha* merge to become SO'HAM, which means "I am That," where "That" refers to the Universal Consciousness. According to the yogis, with every breath we unknowingly affirm the truth "I am That—Universal Consciousness." The *Vijñānabhairavatantra* (verse 156) notes that this silent mantra repeats 21,600 times a day—about 15 times a minute. Thus, our breath becomes japa, a ceaseless chant to the divine, and with it our life becomes a continuous meditative remembrance of our own divine nature.

This silent mantra that we all are spontaneously repeating as we breathe is also known as the *haṁsa* mantra, *haṁsa* meaning "swan," the vehicle of the goddess Sarasvatī—the deity of self-knowledge. Symbolically, the imagery of the goddess Sarasvatī seated on the swan signifies that the knowledge of who we truly are is not somewhere out there; it is always with us—in every breath we take, in every moment we live. We just need to access it through remembrance.

Initially, the practitioner cultivates conscious awareness of SO'HAM with each inhale and exhale. But as the practice deepens, breath and awareness merge into a single, seamless current of remembrance. Over time, the boundaries between inhalation and exhalation, the doer and the observer, and doing and being begin to dissolve, reminding us that the True Self is not somewhere else; it is with us, within us—intimately woven into our very breath. This is one of those rare yogic gifts that is accessible to all, requiring nothing except mindful breaths—where the ordinary act of breathing becomes a gateway to the sacred.

I have personally practiced ajapā in my own sādhanā for over twenty-two years, and it remains one of the most grounding and integrating tools in my daily life. Whether in stillness or in motion, it threads my awareness through the fabric of the day, allowing my breath to serve as a bridge between the outer and the inner, the temporal and the timeless. When I get caught up in the noise of my mind, I simply return to the quiet rhythm of my inner SO'HAM, which is going on relentlessly, no matter what.

Prāṇa Ūrdhvagamana: The Ascending Path

In the context of Tantra, particularly in seminal works like the *Svacchandatantra* (5.68) and Abhinavagupta's *Tantrasāra* (chapter 5), terms such as *udghāta* and *ucchāra*, where *ud* implies an ascent, refer to advanced spiritual processes that involve the conscious elevation of prāṇa and, thereby, one's own awareness. Far beyond ordinary breathwork or chanting, these are refined inner technologies that combine sound (nāda), breath, visualization, and focused awareness to lift the prāṇa upward, purify the subtle body (sūkṣma śarīra), and dissolve entrenched karmic patterns deposited over lifetimes. This energetic ascent is not merely symbolic; it is a lived, vibratory awakening through which the seeker doesn't just experience higher states of consciousness but gradually becomes established in them, culminating in a liberated state (*mokṣa*) of union with the all-pervading reality.

Some advanced yogis, through years of deep inner discipline and mastery over prāṇa, are known to voluntarily withdraw their prāṇa from the body in a deliberate and conscious manner, often directing it upward toward the *brāhmarandhra*—the subtle aperture at the crown of the head. This upward movement of prāṇa is the ascent toward liberation. Texts like the *Haṭha Tattva Kaumudī* (53.1–2) describe this process as the culmination of intense prāṇic regulation and inner absorption.

Maharṣi Patañjali, too, describes the extraordinary possibilities that arise from mastery over udāna. In Yoga Sūtra 3.39, he speaks of the power to levitate, and in 3.38, he alludes to the ability of the mind to enter other bodies (*para-śarīra-āveśa*). Such esoteric abilities, made possible through deep understanding and control of prāṇa, are not just theoretical. They are documented across a wide spectrum of yogic texts and lived through the lives of accomplished yogis and saints throughout the Indian spiritual tradition.

Closely related is the phenomenon of *jīva samādhi*, a state in which an accomplished adept (*jīvanmukta*) consciously enters deep samādhi, withdrawing prāṇa from the physical body, not as an act of dying in the conventional sense but as a self-directed transcendence of bodily existence. In some cases, the physical body is preserved in a sacred, motionless state, believed to remain subtly infused with prāṇic energy. A parallel to this can be found in Tibetan Buddhism in the phenomenon known as *thukdam*, where advanced practitioners remain in a meditative, post-death state for days or even weeks, showing no signs of decomposition, believed to be the result of retained prāṇa and ongoing meditative absorption even after clinical death.

These extraordinary occurrences reflect the immense potential of prāṇa, not merely as a biological force but as a conscious, spiritual energy that can be directed, refined, and ultimately transcended by those who have fully realized its nature.

ENDING INSIGHT

Prāṇa practices in the yogic tradition are vast and nuanced, yet they can be broadly categorized into the following four distinct goals, each illuminating a vital dimension of human growth, integration, and transcendence:

1. **Religiospiritual**: Practices like prāṇa pratiṣṭhā and prāṇa upāsanā reveal prāṇa as a sacred bridge between the human and the divine—a living force that invokes and installs sacred presence both in consecrated forms and within one's own inner awareness.

2. **Ethico-moral**: Prāṇāyāma is a powerful means of moral purification and karmic refinement. As *prāyaścitta* (atonement), it helps neutralize the effects of past actions and loosen the grip of limiting tendencies, gradually

dissolving the subtle impressions (saṃskāras) that sustain suffering and cycles of bondage.

3. **Therapeutic**: Perhaps the most universally relevant goal, the therapeutic value of prāṇāyāma, is now backed by science and well established across modern literature. Studies have shown that breath practices reduce anxiety, depression, and pain; regulate blood pressure and hormonal balance; enhance vagal tone; and improve respiratory, cardiovascular, and neurological health.[17] Techniques like nāḍī śodhana, bhrāmarī, bhastrikā, and ujjāyī are widely practiced across the world, and their benefits are accessible to all, regardless of background or belief. Managing prāṇa also means managing how we live. Lifestyle choices, diet, habits, and mental tendencies all influence the flow of prāṇa. Therefore, cultivating moderation (mitāhāra), mindful living, and inner clarity becomes essential for balancing prāṇa. In this light, therapy through prāṇic well-being is not limited to breath practices alone; it is sustained through a conscious, harmonious way of life.

4. **Liberational**: Ultimately, the highest aim of prāṇic practice lies in mokṣa, spiritual liberation. Through refined methods such as kumbhaka and prāṇa dhāraṇā, the practitioner gradually stills the fluctuations of the mind and transcends the duality of self and other.

Thus, prāṇic practices form a complete spectrum—supporting the devotee, the seeker, the healer, and the transcendental aspirant alike. Whether one uses the practices for clarity, for healing, for purification, or for spiritual awakening, prāṇa remains the sacred thread that connects all beings, in all states. This is the brilliance and compassion of the ancient yogic seers. They wove together the full spectrum of human experience through prāṇic wisdom, offering a path that could heal, empower, and ultimately liberate humanity from within.

PRĀṆĀYĀMA: A WAY OF LIFE

When we begin to recognize the diverse presence of prāṇa—not just in the breath but in digestion, circulation, thought, speech, and emotion—we start to understand that prāṇāyāma is not merely a breathing exercise; it's a way of living. Just as true wellness is not confined only to exercising but also includes food, sleep, rest, and mental clarity, the cultivation of prāṇa also requires attention to our body, mind, thoughts, and lifestyle. How we move, what we eat, how we sleep, the thoughts we entertain, and the emotional atmosphere we live in—all influence the quality, flow, and strength of our prāṇa. When seen this way, prāṇāyāma becomes not something we *do*, but something we *live*, moment by moment.

Reflection Exercise: Prāṇāyāma as a Way of Life

Prāṇāyāma begins as a practice but matures into a way of living—an ongoing sensitivity to how energy moves through every aspect of our day. The following reflection questions invite you to observe the subtle ways your choices, rhythms, and inner states shape the flow of prāṇa in daily life.

- What in your day tends to drain your prāṇa, and what activities, people, or moments nourish and replenish it?
- How do your habits of movement, food, rest, and thinking influence the quality and flow of your breath?
- What might it look like to live prāṇāyāma—not only during formal practice but as a continuous awareness and regulation of prāṇa through the day?

6

Life Lessons from Prāṇa

That which is Truth (*Satya*) rests upon
Strength (*Bala*), and *Prāṇa* is that Strength—
therefore, Truth rests upon *Prāṇa*.
—Bṛhadāraṇyaka Upaniṣad (5.14.4)

In a world increasingly defined by distraction—endless notifications, hurried schedules, and the anxiety of what's next, we often lose touch with the silent connection to others, to nature, and above all, to ourselves. Our attention is scattered, our breath shallow, and our presence fractured. And yet, having traveled through the chapters so far, glimpsing the vast, multidimensional landscape of prāṇa, we may now feel eager to put this understanding into practice. Fortunately, we live in a time where a wide range of breath modalities and prāṇāyāma techniques are easily accessible to us. But before we rush to try different practices, it's worth pausing to remember a deeper truth:

Sometimes, remembrance itself *is* the practice. It is this quiet remembrance—carried in the background of our daily life—that gradually shapes how we breathe, think, and respond. In a world of doing, what we may truly need is *being*—anchored in awareness of what prāṇa is.

FIVE ESSENTIAL TRUTHS

This closing chapter doesn't offer new practices; instead, it provides the following five essential truths about our relationship with prāṇa—truths that, when gently remembered in daily life, help us realign our body, mind, and the flow of life itself:

1. Prāṇa is sacred aliveness.
2. Prāṇa is a dependable partner.
3. Prāṇa is a shared communion.
4. Prāṇa is the compassionate mother.
5. Prāṇa is the leader and teacher.

Prāṇa Is Sacred Aliveness

Prāṇa is something we live and feel every moment—through how we breathe, sense, move, and show up in the world. Each breath is more than just a physical act; it carries our emotions and awareness. As the sage in the *Kauṣītaki Upa-*

niṣad (3.3) declares, "Prāṇa is *prajñā* (self-awareness); and prajñā is prāṇa," pointing to the intimate unity between our breath and our conscious awareness.

When we begin to recognize how closely prāṇa shapes and sustains our life, each inhalation and exhalation becomes a living reminder of the mantra SO'HAM—"I am That." It reminds us that we're not here just to get by or move through life on autopilot but to live with awareness, fullness, and purpose. To truly live with prāṇa is to awaken to life as a sacred, ongoing journey of becoming more alive, more present, and more connected.

Lesson: The world may sometimes weigh us down, test our patience, or blur our sense of purpose. Yet, let every breath remind you that life isn't meant to be merely endured but lived with awareness, lightness, and joy. With each inhale, feel prāṇa as your quiet choice to open to the possibilities around you. Life isn't just happening to you; it's inviting you to dance with it, moment by moment, breath by breath. The science of prāṇa asks us to meet life not mechanically but as a sacred participation in the living flow of life.

Prāṇa Is a Dependable Partner

Prāṇa is in us because we are immersed in it. As wind, food, water, breath, and the subtle workings of our mind and body, it is our constant companion—an unseen partner in every moment of life. It walks with us, fuels our thoughts, powers our movements, helps us respond to emotions, and carries us through every high and low. Together, we shape the prāṇic field that we call our life. Whether we are aware of it or not, prāṇa never abandons us, not even in death. This partnership has been deeply emphasized by the ṛṣis, as expressed in the *Bṛhadāraṇyaka Upaniṣad* (3.7.2), which declares: "*Prāṇa* (vāyu) is the thread (sūtra) by which all beings are held together—through this life and the next."

When we live with awareness of this truth, we begin to realize that we are not alone—we never were. In prāṇa we have a partner who adapts, empowers, heals, and responds—someone who works *with* us, *as* us. To live with this ever-faithful prāṇa partner is to learn to trust—trust life as it comes. From prāṇa, we also learn resilience, adaptability, and lasting commitment. It reminds us to keep going, to rest when we need to, to act with awareness, and to keep finding our way back to balance—just like an easy, natural breath. When we truly recognize prāṇa as our partner and commit to the partnership, we find the inspiration to live more consciously and be our best—without fear, without doubt, knowing we are never alone. Together, moment by moment, *we two keep shaping life as we go.*

Lesson: As you live your day, pause and sense the presence of prāṇa moving with you—walking, resting, rising, and falling like a faithful companion. Let this awareness remind you that you are never alone or abandoned; every step you take is supported by the subtle thread of life that never leaves your side.

Prāṇa Is a Shared Communion

Our breathing is not just a purely personal act; it is a shared responsibility, a collective rhythm that binds all living beings. With every inhale and exhale, we draw from and return to the same atmosphere that sustains all of life—trees, animals, oceans, and humans alike. The air we breathe today has been circulating through Earth's ecosystems for billions of years, moving through countless lungs, both human and nonhuman, across time. We are not merely inhaling molecules; we are participating in a vast, ongoing dance of life's shared breath. The water we drink has journeyed through ancient rivers, clouds, and bodies. Even the food we eat carries within it the quiet memory of space and time. In every act of nourishment, we are woven into a shared, ongoing story of survival. In this way, prāṇa is not simply our own; it is a sacred communion, a thread that weaves us into the living fabric of existence. As the *Muṇḍaka Upaniṣad* (3.1.4) states, prāṇa shines variously within all living beings.

To live with awareness of this communion is to live with reverence—for our life, for the life of others, and for the planet that holds us all. Recognizing prāṇa as a shared reality invites us to breathe, eat, live, and consume natural resources not just mindfully, but responsibly. Each breath is a reminder that we are not isolated beings but part of a vast, intelligent, and interdependent whole. We breathe as one, but we live for all.

Lesson: With every breath, pause to sense the greater whole you belong to—the forests, rivers, skies, and beings that breathe with you. Let this awareness touch the way you live with more care, more reverence, knowing that everything you do sends ripples through the shared breath of life.

Prāṇa Is the Compassionate Mother

Prāṇa is revered across the yogic traditions as a mother, Prāṇa Śakti—the protector and the provider of all life. She takes many sacred forms, each embodying a facet of her boundless care. As Kuṇḍalinī Śakti, she is the very source of our individuality, guarding our deepest human potential and gradually unfolding it with grace. As Bhūmi Devī, she becomes the earth beneath our feet—holding us and offering food, shelter, and grounding. As Prakṛti, the manifested existence, she is the ever-giving matrix of form and function. As Mātā Sarasvatī, the goddess of wisdom, she rides on the swan of breath—the haṃsa, reminding us that true knowledge is carried on the wings of every single inhale and exhale.

As the power behind movement, creation, and sustenance, she nourishes not just our limbs and lungs, but also our decisions and dreams. Like a responsible mother, she watches over us—protecting through her energies, supporting through her gifts, giving without asking, and upholding us even when we forget her presence. As the prayer in the *Praśna Upaniṣad* (2.13) tenderly invokes, "O Prāṇa, protect us as a mother protects her children. Bless us with prosperity and wisdom."

To remember prāṇa as Śakti, the compassionate mother, is to feel supported by a presence greater than ourselves—one that nourishes, guides, and protects. She invites us to live with reverence, embodying her strength and care. In honoring her, we learn to live not just more wisely but more tenderly.

Lesson: With every breath, remember you are held by a caring higher intelligence. Allow yourself to rest in its support, receive its care, and move through life with gratitude.

Prāṇa Is the Leader and Teacher

One may dismiss breath as ordinary, mundane, and too subtle to notice, yet in its quiet working lies one of our greatest teachers. Prāṇa, expressed through breath, does not merely keep us alive; it leads, nurtures, and educates us. When our mind is scattered, it takes over, breathing for us without demand. But the moment we become conscious of our breath, our body, our choices—it steps aside and lets us lead. In this way, prāṇa is the ideal leader: supportive when we falter, empowering as we rise. It neither dominates nor abandons; it accompanies us with intelligence and grace. Like a true leader, it doesn't just guide; it trusts us to grow into our own power.

Our breath cycles are not linear. They move in spirals of expansion and return, echoing the rhythm of the Moon, the tides, and the heartbeat of life. Between each inhale and exhale lies a pause that reflects those gentle spaces where the mind softens and awareness deepens. In those spaces prāṇa teaches us the power of stillness—the wisdom of waiting, the clarity that comes from listening before speaking, and the sophistication of reflecting before reacting. Like a compassionate teacher, it watches the mind with patience, allowing our awareness to ripen in its own time. It does not demand or dominate; it simply stays constant, faithful, and ready. In that steady assurance, we find our rightful place in the greater whole. As the *Chāndogya Upaniṣad* (7.15.1) reverently affirms, prāṇa is the *ācārya*—the teacher who leads not through instruction alone but through the silent inspiration of its own presence and workings.

Thus, prāṇa is the original guru—gentle yet relentless,

invisible yet ever-present, holding our hand through each inhale of hope and exhale of release, guiding us through the dualities of life. To recognize prāṇa as the guru is to trust that each breath carries the guidance we need to return to ourselves.

Lesson: True guidance empowers, not controls. With every breath, let yourself be guided as prāṇa teaches—rest in its stillness, trust its rhythm, and know that life itself will bring the moments you need to grow, learn, and awaken the wisdom within. And when doubt arises, gently remind yourself that you are being guided, always—as surely as each breath.

ENDING INSIGHT

Breath is the universe quietly flowing through us. We are part of one vast, living flow. The same breath that sustains us also stirs the stars and holds all of life together. To breathe consciously is to remember this connection—to align ourselves with the deeper current that links our inner and outer worlds. When we begin to sense prāṇa not just as a bodily function but as a living presence, we rediscover our place in the larger harmony of life.

In Sanskrit, the word for trust and confidence is *viśvāsa*—composed of *vi* (special) and *śvāsa* (breath or life). Trust and confidence, then, quite literally mean "a special breath."

Your trust—your confidence—is a special breath. Isn't that beautiful? It suggests that true confidence, sincere trust is not forced from the mind but arises naturally from a steady, open breath.

We've all felt it—that breath of confidence that comes when we feel calm. A breath that is grounded in trust, reminding us that life is supporting us, that we can lean in and let go just a little more. It's full, deep, and satisfying. Every single breath matters. Each breath is part of an unbroken continuum that quietly shapes our body, mind, and the quality of our life. The state of our mind, body, and life begins with how we breathe. Each conscious breath is a quiet act of trust—a way of saying yes to life again, with steadiness and ease.

For the ancient ṛṣis, every breath and every interaction with prāṇa was a way to stay attuned to the sacred rhythm of existence. May this understanding inspire us to breathe with greater depth and live with gentle reverence for the life force that moves through us all. In a world that can often feel heavy and unpredictable, we can remember the quiet truth the ṛṣis handed down: Life itself is sacred, our breath is a bridge, and prāṇa has the power to uplift not only our own being but the shared fabric of human experience. This is how we live the ancient wisdom of prāṇa—by knowing it, by breathing it, by being it, and by becoming it. Through the mindful harmony of body, mind, and breath, we begin to sense prāṇa not merely as energy but as the conscious force uniting all aspects of our existence—a subtle strand running through and connecting every level of our being, reminding us to live in rhythm with the intelligence that breathes through all.

Notes

1. *Aṣṭādhyāyī* 8.4.19 in Sumitra M. Katre, trans., *Aṣṭādhyāyī of Pāṇini in Roman Transliteration* (University of Texas Press, 1987).
2. Swami Gambhirananda, trans., *Eight Upanishads: With the Commentary of Sankaracarya* (Advaita Ashrama, 1989), 434.
3. Christian Mütze, Dietmar Mitzinger, and Heidemarie Haller, "Effectiveness of Pranayama for Mental Disorders: A Systematic Review and Meta-Analysis of Randomized Controlled Trials," *Frontiers in Psychiatry* 16 (2025). This study showed that prāṇāyāma significantly reduced post-intervention symptom severity in comparison to passive controls in patients with PTSD, depression, and mixed nonpsychotic mental disorders.
4. J. B. West and A. Luks, *West's Respiratory Physiology: The Essentials*, 10th ed. (Wolters Kluwer, 2016); A. B. Lumb *Nunn's Applied Respiratory Physiology*, 8th ed. (Elsevier, 2017).
5. W. N. Gardner, "The Pathophysiology of Hyperventilation Disorders." *Chest* 109, no. 2 (1996): 516–34.
6. Eric R. Kandel et al., *Principles of Neural Science*, 5th ed. (McGraw-Hill Education, 2014).
7. Rollin McCraty and Doc Childre, "Coherence: Bridging Personal, Social, and Global Health," *Alternative Therapies in Health and Medicine* 16, no. 4 (2010): 10–24.

8. Centers for Disease Control and Prevention. *Digital Technology and Mental Health in Teens* (U.S. Department of Health & Human Services, 2024).
9. E. J. Zampella et al., "The Role of Oxidative Stress in Chronic Respiratory Diseases," *Antioxidants*, no. 8 (2018): 110.
10. T. Soroka et al., "Humans Have Nasal Respiratory Fingerprints," *Current Biology* 35, no. 13 (June 12, 2025), www.cell.com/current-biology/fulltext/S0960-9822(25)00583-4.
11. The *Jñānēśvarī* is a comprehensive commentary on the *Bhagavad Gītā* composed in 1290 C.E. by the Marathi saint and realized Haṭha Yoga and Bhakti master Sant Jñānēśwar.
12. M. Huang et al., "Healthy Lifestyle and Cardiac Vagal Modulation Over 10 Years: Whitehall II Cohort Study," *Journal of the American Heart Association* 8, no. 19.
13. James Mallinson and Mark Singleton, *Roots of Yoga* (Penguin Classics, 2017), 140.
14. P. M. Lehrer and R. Gevirtz, "Heart Rate Variability Biofeedback: How and Why Does It Work?" *Frontiers in Psychology* 5 (2014): 756. (This article explores the mechanism, particularly the role of resonance breathing in boosting heart rate variability and vagal function.)
15. R. Jerath et al., "Physiology of Long Pranayamic Breathing: Neural Respiratory Elements May Provide a Mechanism that Explains How Slow Deep Breathing Shifts the Autonomic Nervous System," *Medical Hypotheses* 67, no. 3 (2006): 566–71. https://doi.org/10.1016/j.mehy.2006.02.042.
16. J. Annen et al., "Mapping the Functional Brain State of a World Champion Freediver in Static Dry Apnea," *Experimental Brain Research* 239, no. 11 (2021): 3163–75.
17. R. P. Brown and P. L. Gerbarg Sudarshan, "Kriya Yogic Breathing in the Treatment of Stress, Anxiety, and Depression. Part II—Clinical Applications and Guidelines," *Journal*

of Alternative and Complementary Medicine 11, no. 4 (2005): 711–17; R. Jerath, "Physiology of Long Pranayamic Breathing: Neural Respiratory Elements May Provide a Mechanism That Explains the Benefits of Slow Deep Breathing," *Medical Hypotheses* 67, no. 3 (2006): 566–71.